The S

MW01233075

Step-by-Step Beginners Guide to Lose Weight Quickly and Improve Your Health.

Discover the amazing benefits of sirt foods to loose over then 7 lbs in the first week.

Includes 31 Delicious Recipes and a 7-day Meal Plan.

STEVEN FUNG

Copyright © 2020 Steven Fung

Table of Contents

Olive Oil
Garlic
Green Tea
Kale
Medjool Dates
Parsley
Red Endive
Red Onion
Soy
Red Wine
Strawberries
Turmeric
Walnut

Sirtuins
Sirtuins Present In Human Beings
Sirtfood Diet

Tips For Sticking To Your Diet Plan

Starting With Expectations That Are Real
Thinking About All Those Things That Can
Motivate You
Keeping Food Items Out Of Reach That Is Not
Included In The Plan
Not Having All Or Nothing Kind Of Approach

Carrying Healthy Snacks
Exercising And Changing The Diet At Same Point
Having A Game Plan Before Consuming Food
Do Not Allow Your Travelling Schedule To Derail
You
Practicing Mindful Eating
Tracking And Monitoring The Progress
Getting A Partner For Joining You
Realizing That It Will Take Time For Changing The
Habits
Figuring Out What Will Work Out The Best

Turning The Diet In Your Daily Lifestyle

Exercising After The Diet
Importance Of Exercising

Can Give You A Happy Feeling
Exercising And Weight Loss
Exercising Is Beneficial For The Bones And Muscles
Improvement Of Energy Levels
Exercise Can Reduce Chronic Diseases
Improves Skin Health
Improve Brain Memory And Health
Exercise Can Improve The Quality Of Sleep
Exercise Can Help In Reducing Pain

Can I Exercise During The First Phase Of The Diet?
Can I Opt For Sirtdiet If I Am Underweight Or
Excessively Thin?
Can I Stop Following The Diet After Achieving The
Target Body Weight?
Can I Stop Drinking The Green Juice After
Completing The Second Phase Of The Diet?
Can I Follow The Sirtdiet While Taking Medicinal
Drugs?
Can I Follow The Diet At The Time Of Pregnancy?
How Frequently Can I Opt For The Phases Of The
Diet?

INTRODUCTION

Congratulations on purchasing *The Sirtfood Diet,* and thank you for doing so.

In this world of new trends every day, new diets also pop up daily. Sirtfood diet is among one of the new diet plans that are trending today. 'Sirtfoods' are regarded as the secret key for unlocking loss of fat and also for preventing various diseases. Most of the dieticians recommend sirtfood diet as a healthy and revolutionary diet plan that functions by turning on the 'skinny gene.' The diet is based on several types of research on SIRTs or sirtuins, a small group of seven beneficial proteins that are found in the body. This group of proteins can easily regulate various functions of the body, such as inflammation, metabolism, and lifespan.

This book is all about the basics of sirtfood diet along with several recipes that can help you in your journey. After you are done with the complete diet, you will feel encouraged to include sirtfoods in your daily diet plan. According to the creators of sirtfood diet, it can help in losing weight rapidly while maintaining the muscle mass and also overall protection from various chronic diseases. The diet involves calorie restriction as well, which makes it even more effective. You will need to follow certain meal plans that will help you with the diet.

There are plenty of books on this subject on the market, thanks again for choosing this one! Every effort was made to ensure it is full of as much useful information as possible; please enjoy!

CHAPTER 1: INTRODUCTION TO SIRTFOOD DIET

Sirtfood diet can be regarded as a new member of the diet world that was designed and developed by two nutritionists from the United Kingdom. The developers of the diet started marketing the diet as the 'revolution of diet.' It was even marketed as an effective health strategy that can work very easily by turning on the skinny gene in the system of the human body.

What Is Sirtfood Diet?

The sirtfood diet is the trendiest way of burning body fat and also lose bodyweight without even experiencing starving or malnutrition. Activation of the skinny gene is done with the help of fasting and exercising. There are certain food categories that come with chemicals called polyphenols. Polyphenols, when consumed, can put a bit of stress on the cells of the human body. This results in the production of the genes that can follow the consequences of exercising and fasting. Such food items include red wine, chocolate, coffee, kale, and others. As you consume any food items of this kind, they will be releasing sirtuins that can influence mood swings, aging, and even metabolism of the body. Any form of diet that is rich in sirtuins can trigger weight loss with no need to expend the body muscles. You will also be leading a healthy body and lifestyle at the same point in time.

Sirtfood diet is focused particularly on the restriction of calories that is done in different phases. This form of calorie restriction can help in improving sirtuin production in the human body. Many people often think whether the diet is good for them or not. Well, each and every food items that are included in the plan of diet are extremely healthy. You will be getting the perfect number of vitamins, nutrients, and minerals that will considerably improve as you follow the diet properly. However, this particular diet is a bit restrictive in nature for certain types of foods, along with calories. So, it might turn out to be a bit tough for certain people to get accustomed to the same and follow it.

Effectiveness Of Sirtfood Diet

The developers of this diet are very positive about the effectiveness of the diet for weight loss, for burning fat, for activating the skinny gene, and for inhibiting various concerns related to health. But, there is very little evidence for backing these. There is no sudden proof that can ascertain the positive effects of this diet on the human body when compared to other diets of calorie restriction. All the foods that are included in this diet are full of nutrients, vitamins, and minerals. But, there is no study regarding the health benefits of being on a diet that is rich in sirtfoods.

The key to this diet is that you will need to follow the diet until you reach the desired goal and then maintain the same. You will need to maintain it strictly for getting the most out of it. When your body experiences deprivation of energy, it will start utilizing the stored form of emergency energy or glycogen. This, in turn, will result in the burning of fat. In short, a sirtfood diet can help you in losing weight as it is low in calorie count. But, you will need to prepare yourself for maintaining the same as once the diet gets over, you will be gaining weight again. The primary reason behind this is that the diet is short in nature for having long term effects on the body.

The Skinny Gene

The majority of the people in this world are not happy with the shape of their body, and they find their size unappealing and unattractive; this results in feeling disturbed about the ways in which we can contour, control, and change the shape of our body. We all have come across people in our lives who cannot gain weight no matter how much food they consume. Several research and studies have been done to find out how certain people do not seem to gain any extra pounds taking into consideration their way of eating, while other people gain a lot of weight excessively. The answer to this can be found in the genes. There is nothing as a perfect gene. While discussing obesity and weight gain, genetics is something that we must take into consideration. Genetics can play a deep role in gaining weight and obesity as well.

Some people come with the blessing of the skinny gene, and they can activate the same while others cannot. Even if you belong to the unlucky group, there are certain things that can be done on your part for turning on and off the gene that you want to. Well, it might sound funny but it is possible with the secret of gene interaction. It is the process that is involved with the task of improving the way in which the genes interact with the environment.

Sirtuins or the skinny gene functions very actively in altering the way in which the cells function. Sirtuins are very effective for burning body fat. They are considered special in nature as they come with the capability of turning the body cells in a mode of survival. This whole thing is done with the help of a process that is known as autophagy. Autophagy is also responsible for getting rid of wastes of the cells along with various unwanted particles that get piled up with time. Storing up unwanted particles can result in inflammation. The result of the restoration process is actually alarming in nature– it makes the cells of the body look younger, makes them healthy, and reduces inflammation. Activation of this gene is the key that helps in initiating loss of weight and also leads to the prevention of various issues related to health.

Activating Compounds

Certain food items can effectively activate the skinny gene or sirtuins in our bodies. But, the perfect amount of such food items that are required for activating the sirtuin is still unknown. The activators elevate the sensitivity to insulin and also reduce the level of blood sugar to a great extent. Let's have a look at some of the activators.

- **Polyphenols:** Can be found in turmeric. A little amount is required for having positive effects on the human body. In case you consume it in high amounts, it might turn out to be dangerous.

- **Quercetin:** It can be found in kale, apple, capers, onion, citrus fruits, and berries. It can help in dealing with inflammation.

- **Resveratrol:** You can find this in raspberries, peanuts, and blueberries. It can help in improving the health of the heart and also deals with inflammation.

- **Piceatannol**: It is used as an herbal-grade medicine in the countries of Asia. It can be found in red and white wine.

- **Fisetin**: It can be found in strawberries and can help in improving memory of long term.

- **Oligonol**: Can be found in litchi. It is rich in properties that can deal with inflammation.

- **Omega-3**: It can be found in salmon, tilapia, catfish, and flaxseeds.

As you consume food source of any of the mentioned activating compounds, it can help in activating sirtuin proteins in the body. There are certainly other ways as well that can help in turning on the skinny gene, and that is with the help of exercise and fasting. Although it might sound very simple, it is quite difficult for several people taking into consideration the busy type of schedule that leaves no time for fasting or exercising. After the result of fasting is a feeling of anger and hunger that can result in the stagnation of body metabolism. While discussing exercising, the intensity of exercise that is needed for losing weight relies on the effort and strength that has been given in.

The Weight Gain Genes

There are genes that can be linked to weight gain. Such genes include:

FTO Gene

FTO gene or fat mass and obesity gene is regarded as having the strongest connection with the index of body mass. It is the greatest risk of developing obesity and diabetes. There is a specific variant that helps in turning on the gene. If that variant is there in the body, you will have no control over the satiety hormone that is known as leptin. This can result in making you consume food without any reason. This gene tends to function as a sensor of fat. People who come with this gene in their body have the tendency to eat unnecessarily and excessively, specifically fatty foods. People who come with an abnormal nature of genes from their parents tend to have more weight and have the risk of developing obesity. People with normal genes are at a lower risk of developing obesity.

The FTO gene gets turned on with the proper and adequate exercise. You will need to ensure that you sleep for 7 – 8 hours, consume food that comes with low carbohydrate and increase the intake of fiber. As you follow a good lifestyle and proper diet, you can effectively reduce the risk of developing obesity.

Melanocortin 4 Receptor

People who come with this gene will tend to have more

amounts of snacks, even when they are not feeling hungry. Such people are most likely to spend their time snacking on chips, cake, and others. In short, this gene can increase the overall urge to consume fat. In case you have the urge to snack, try to have three meals in a day. Set the meal routine at a gap of six to seven hours between the meals and try not to touch any kind of snacks in between.

Gut Bacteria And Its Role In Genes

According to the studies conducted with gut bacteria, several results have showcased the existence of certain bacteria that can be linked with body weight. The only thing that is known is that such bacteria results in the production of certain chemicals that can bring about certain changes in the genes of people. Gut bacteria can show their influence right from the time of birth. Babies who are born from cesarean have been found to have a balance of a different kind when compared with babies who are born naturally. There are certain steps that can be taken to enhance the health of gut bacteria, stimulating body weight.

Nutrition For Turning On And Off The Genes

It is true that the type of food that we consume and the environment in which we tend to live can have some significant nature of effects on the genetic makeup. The sirtuins or skinny gene is believed to exist in all of us, and we just need to find out the same and switch it on. Certain people may be exposed to specific things because of the makeup of their genes in relation to the weight of their body and various other factors. Genes can be overcome actually in case it is the primary reason behind increasing body weight. When done in the proper way, you will be able to lose the weight that is causing all the trouble.

However, there is no possible reason behind blaming your genetic makeup for your obesity. As already mentioned earlier, genes tend to play only a 10 – 15% role in developing obesity, and the rest is the result of the factors of the environment. You will need to make necessary adjustments wherever needed without blaming the genes for the problem of being overweight. One such way is by following the sirtfood diet that can help in losing weight without any kind of adverse effects on the muscle mass. There are certain foods that you will need to include in your diet. All of that will be discussed in the upcoming chapters.

CHAPTER 2: BENEFITS OF SIRTFOOD DIET

Sirtfood diet involves various types of food items that you can enjoy while being on a diet as well. Some of the food items include dark chocolate, red wine, strawberries, and so on. The main goal of a sirtfood diet is to restrict calorie intake that can trigger the system of the body to produce higher levels of sirtuins.

It has been found that during the starting of the diet plan, you can lose about 3 kgs during the first week.

You will also be able to notice a change in the levels of your energy, quality of the skin, and your sleep quality as well. According to the creators of the sirtfood diet, sirtfoods can help in satiating and increasing the function of the body muscles. This will help you to achieve better and healthy body weight. In fact, the benefits of this diet are considered to be more beneficial when compared to some of the chronic drugs. Also, it has been said that a sirtfood diet can help in treating people who are suffering from Alzheimer's disease. No one can deny that sirtfoods are good for human health. They are full of healthy compounds and are also rich in nutrient content.

For example, if you consume a little amount of dark chocolate that comes with a high content of cocoa, it can help in lowering the overall risk of developing heart diseases. It can also help in dealing with inflammation. Also, if you drink green tea, it can lower the risk of diabetes and stroke. It will also help in maintaining proper blood pressure. In fact, most of the foods that are included in the sirtfood diet have shown health-related benefits.

Several types of research have demonstrated that a higher level of sirtuin in the body can help in improving the lifespan of worms, mice, and yeast. During calorie restriction or fasting, the sirtuin proteins indicate the body to burn out more amount of fat for producing energy and thus improve sensitivity to insulin. Although studies in human and mice cells have depicted positive results, no study has been conducted for examining the overall effect of a higher level of sirtuins in the body. Thus, whether higher levels of sirtuin protein in the body will lower the risk of developing cancer or will help in improving the lifespan is not yet known.

Is Sirtfood Diet Sustainable And Healthy?

Sirtfoods are mostly healthy in nature and can result in certain health benefits because of anti-inflammation or antioxidant properties. However, consuming only a handful of certain healthy foods will not be able to meet all the nutritional requirements of the body. You will need to drink three green juices every day. It is true that green juice is a great source of minerals and vitamins. They are also a great sugar source. But, because of the low level of calories along with restrictive choices of food, sirtfood diet might turn out to be a tough one to stick to for three entire weeks.

Side Effects And Safety

It is true that the first phase of the diet is low in calorie count and is incomplete from the perspective of nutrients. But, there are no forms of safety concerns for the healthy average adults because of the short duration of the diet. However, for people who are suffering from diabetes, restricting calories and living mainly on juice for the first section of the diet might result in some serious changes in the level of blood sugar. Not only that, but a healthy adult can also suffer from a definite side effect, and that is hunger. However, fasting and feeling hungry is the aim of this diet. Having only 1500 – 1600 calories every day can leave any human being feeling very hungry, specifically if you are living only on juices that are low in fiber. This is because fiber is responsible for making you feel full. During the first phase of the diet, you might also suffer from some other side effects like irritability, fatigue, and lightheadedness because of the restricting level of calories.

The sirtfood diet is full of healthy foods but not any definite pattern of eating. But, you can still add some of the sirtfoods to your daily diet for getting a hold of the whole thing before you jump in for the actual diet.

There is a definite routine for the diet that you will need to follow to get the most out of the diet. The phases of the sirtfood diet will be discussed in the later chapters of the book.

CHAPTER 3: WHAT ARE THE SIRTFOODS?

There are various food items that can be included in your plan of sirtfood diet. This chapter is all about the various types of sirtfoods that you should include in the diet for getting the most out of the same.

Buckwheat

Flour that is made from buckwheat helps a lot in losing weight. The overall fat content of buckwheat is very low. In fact, the calorie count is less from normal rice or wheat. As the flour comes with a low amount of saturated form of fat, it can stop you from binge-eating or eating unnecessarily. So, it can help in facilitating and maintaining quick digestion. Because of the low amount of fat along with a greater quantity of minerals, it can facilitate controlling diabetes of type II. Not only that, but you can also consume this flour as a superb source of protein that can help you building and maintaining your muscle mass. It will keep the muscle mass in place while will keep the body weight under check as well.

Buckwheat flour is also rich in fiber that can help in improving the process of digestion by lowering down the secretion of bile. It also participates in detoxification of the body by binding up the toxins and excretes them. Thus, if you include this flour in the diet in place of the normal one, it can readily help you in losing a lot of weight.

Arugula

Arugula is a great sirtfood vegetable and is low in calories. It will not only help you to lose weight but also comes with several healthy properties. Arugula is rich in chlorophyll that can help in preventing DNA and liver damage resulting from aflatoxins. For getting the best from the arugula, it is always recommended to consume this vegetable in its raw state. It is composed of 95% water, and thus it can also act as a cooling and hydrating food for the summer days. Vitamin K plays an important role in maintaining bone health. It is also required for calcium absorption in the teeth and bones. One cup of arugula can provide you with 10.8 micrograms of vitamin K. If you can consume two to three cups of this vegetable every day, you can provide the body with the required percentage of vitamin K.

Arugula is rich in fiber, and it can help in cleaning out

the colon for promoting healthy movements of the bowel. It also participates in detoxification of the body with the help of its antioxidants and phytochemicals. Arugula is rich in vitamin B. If you include arugula in your daily diet, it can provide you with various nutrients. The best part about arugula is that two cups of it contains only about 80 calories, thus making this veggie a great choice for losing weight. Arugula contains glucosinolates that have shown effective results in reducing the overall risk of developing prostate, lung, pancreatic, and breast cancer. Thus, arugula can be regarded as the master of the sirtfood group.

Capers

Caper is the unripe flower bud of Capparis spinosa. Every 100 grams of this contains only 24 calories and thus making it a great companion for losing weight. It is rich in compounds of flavonoid that also includes quercetin and rutin. Both compounds are great sources of antioxidants. Antioxidants can act readily in preventing free radicals that can lead to skin diseases and also cancer. Capers can help in keeping a check on diabetes. It contains several chemicals that can keep the level of blood sugar under control. Capers are also regarded as the mineral mine as it contains minerals such as copper, calcium, iron, and also great quantities of sodium. Calcium can help in building up strong bone structure along with string teeth. Iron helps in storing and using oxygen in the body muscles.

Capers can help by aiding in the excretion of fluids from the body and thus relieve the body from swelling. It comes with a choleretic effect that can help in the digestion process and also makes the food perfectly tasty. In case you are suffering from constipation, capers can help you with that as well. It is a great source of fiber as one tablespoon of it contains about 0.4 g of fiber. People who love to include red meat and other fats in their daily diet can include capers as it helps in destroying several byproducts that can be found in fat–rich foods and meats.

Chilies

Well, this might sound a bit bizarre, but chilies can actually help in losing weight. Consumption of chilies in your daily diet can help in burning down calories. So, adding a bit of spice to your daily diet can help in getting rid of the extra calories and thus can also help in boosting up the metabolism. According to the weight loss experts, cayenne pepper infused with water can have positive effects on the body along with weight loss. A substance, known as capsaicin, can be found in chilies that provides the heat. This can help in preventing weight gain along with obesity as the intake of calories is very less. It also helps in lowering the levels of blood fat. It has also been found that people who have the habit of consuming red pepper in their diet can feel full easily, and thus, it can lower your food cravings.

As chilies participate in boosting body metabolism, the increased rate of metabolism participates in speeding up the ability of the body to convert beverages and food into useful energy. As the metabolism turns out to be faster, the body will be able to convert the important nature of nutrients into useful energy and will also aid in fat burning. You can include chilies in your daily diet, but make sure that you consume it moderately. Capsaicin also comes with properties of anti-inflammation.

Celery

One large stalk of celery contains about 10 calories every hundred grams and that is more than enough for losing weight. It can also aid in preventing dehydration as celery comes with a great amount of water and electrolytes that also helps in lowering the rate of bloating. It comes with antiseptic properties and prevents various problems of the kidney. Consumption of this vegetable can also help in excreting toxic elements from the body. Celery comes with great amounts of vitamin K and vitamin C, along with potassium and folate. It has been found that celery can help in preventing liver diseases, along with cancer. It can also help in boosting the health of the cardiovascular system and also aids in reducing inflammation.

Cocoa

Intake of cocoa, even in its chocolate form, can help in controlling weight. Cocoa comes along with fat-burning properties and is the prime reason why most of the trainers suggest mixing cocoa in shakes before exercising. It can help in reducing inflammation and thus can also help in proper digestion. Cocoa is rich in antioxidants like polyphenols. It can provide you with various health benefits like a better flow of blood, lower level of blood pressure, and also controlled levels of blood sugar. Cocoa, when consumed in the form of chocolate or in its powdered form, can help in aiding high blood pressure.

Cocoa comes with flavanols that can improve the levels of nitric oxide in the blood. It can also help in improving the functioning of the brain. It is true that overconsumption of cocoa is not a good thing for your health; it does come with certain anti-diabetic properties. It has been found that cocoa can help in improving the secretion of insulin, stimulates the process of up taking sugar out of the stream of blood into the body muscles, and also reduces inflammation. Cocoa powder can also help in dealing with stress and has shown positive results in improving the mood.

Coffee

Coffee is one of the most famous beverages that can

be found all over the world. Coffee comes with a very low-calorie count. If you are trying to lose weight, you will need to create a deficit of calories. You can do this by replacing one cup of sweetened beverages with one cup of black coffee. One full cup of brewed coffee comes with only two calories. Caffeine is a form of natural stimulant that is abundant in coffee. Caffeine can help in improving metabolism and thus can act as a great weight loss component. But, you will need to ensure that you consume coffee in a regulated limit; it can affect your sleeping patterns.

Olive Oil

Olive oil has always been a popular medium for cooking food. Olive oil that is of the extra virgin category can help you in losing weight as it is unrefined and unprocessed. It comes with a great percentage of fatty acids of mono-saturated type that plays an important role in losing weight. Olive oil is also rich in vitamin E that is good for the health of hair and skin. It comes with great properties of anti-inflammation as well. Olive oil helps in aiding low absorption of fat and thus makes your food healthy and tasty at the same time. It comes with oleic acid that can retain the important anti-oxidants. It will be easier for you to maintain a healthy heart with proper regulation of the levels of blood sugar. Olive oil comes along with the healthy nature of fats that make it better than any other type of cooking oil.

It can also aid in proper movement of the bowel and can also help in making the health of the gut better.

Garlic

Garlic is one of those vegetables that can be found in every kitchen. It is full of nutrients and also aids in losing weight. Consumption of raw garlic can help in boosting energy levels that can aid in losing weight. Garlic is well known for suppressing appetite that can help you in staying full for more amount of time. Thus, with the consumption of garlic, you will be able to prevent yourself from overeating. A strong relationship can be found between burning fat and the consumption of garlic. Garlic helps in stimulating the process of fat burning and also helps in removing harmful toxins from the body. Thus, it can be said that garlic helps in improving the process of digestion as well. It also comes with several other important elements like vitamin C, vitamin B6, protein, calcium, manganese, and others. This is the primary reason why garlic is regarded as the powerhouse of nutrients.

It comes with antioxidant properties and helps in boosting the immune system. Garlic contains sulfur that can help in stimulating the production of nitric oxide in the blood vessels. It also plays an important role in detoxifying the liver with the help of selenium. So, besides adding taste to your food, garlic can aid in losing weight as well.

Green Tea

Green tea is often regarded as the healthiest type of beverage that can be found on this planet. This is mainly because green tea is full of antioxidants, along with several other plant compounds that can provide you with several health benefits. Green tea consists of caffeine. It can be found in coffee as well and acts as a stimulant for burning fat. It can also help in boosting your levels of energy at the time of exercising. Green tea comes with a high concentration of minerals and vitamins, along with low content of calories. It can help in improving the metabolic rate as well.

Green tea comes along with an ingredient named theanine. It is a form of amino acid that can help in reducing stress by providing effects of relaxation and calmness without any form of sedation. This can help in cutting down excess weight easily. Norepinephrine is a compound that helps in boosting the burning of fat. It is possible to break down fat only when the fat cells are moved to the bloodstream. This whole process is aided by this compound. Include green tea in your daily diet, and you will be able to notice the changes readily.

Kale

Kale is a very popular vegetable that comes with excellent weight loss properties. It is a vegetable that is rich in antioxidants. Kale comes with vitamin C that performs various important functions in the body cells, along with improving the bone structure of the body. It is rich in vitamin K and comes with excellent capabilities of binding calcium. Kale can provide you with 2.4 g of dietary fiber and thus can help in reducing the feeling of hunger. It comes with compounds rich in sulfur and can help in detoxifying the liver.

Medjool Dates

Dates are often linked with increasing weight as they are rich in sugar content. However, according to some recent studies, it has been found that dates can readily help in shedding the extra weight. Dates are rich in dietary fibers along with fatty acids that can help in losing the extra kilos when consumed under moderation. You will be able to stay healthy and fit as dates can provide you with a great deal of protein. Consumption of dates daily can help in boosting the functioning of the immune system.

Parsley

Parsley is a very common herb that can be found in every kitchen. Parsley leaves are low in calorie count. The leaves are rich in important compounds such as vitamin A, vitamin b, vitamin C, and vitamin K. Important minerals such as potassium and iron can also be found in parsley. As it acts as a natural form of diuretic, it can help in flushing out toxins along with any excess fluid. Parsley is rich in chlorophyll, and it can effectively aid in losing weight. It also helps in keeping the levels of blood sugar under control. Parsley comes with certain enzymes that can help in improving the process of digestion and also helps in weight loss.

Red Endive

Endives are rich in fiber with a low-calorie count. It comes with a great combination of elements that can help in promoting weight loss. There is nothing tougher than persistent hunger at the time of losing weight. Endives are rich in fiber that can help in slowing down the process of digestion and keeps the level of energy stable. As red endives are high in water and fiber content, you will be able to consume more volume of food without the risk of consuming extra calories. It is rich in potassium and folate as well that is important for the proper health of the heart. Potassium can act very well in lowering the level of blood pressure. Fiber can also help in improving the profiles of lipids by getting attached to blood cholesterol and then remove the same for excretion.

Folate can aid in protecting the arteries by reducing the risk of heart attack and stroke. Red endives also come with beta carotene and vitamin A that are essential for good vision. Make sure that you include red endives in your diet if you are willing to lose weight fast without any effect on your muscle mass.

Red Onion

Red onion is rich in an antioxidant named quercetin. Red onions can help in adding extra flavor to your food without piling up extra calories. Quercetin helps in promoting burning down extra calories. It can also help in dealing with inflammation. Red onion is rich in fiber and thus can make you feel full for a long period without the urge to consume extra calories. It can also help in improving the level of blood sugar and can deal with diabetes of type II.

Soy

It has been found that increasing the consumption of soy can help in reducing your body weight. It is rich in fiber that can help you to stay full for long. Soy comes along with the essential amino acids that can help in losing weight readily. Soy can also help in regulating the level of blood sugar and can have great control over the appetite. It can also promote better quality skin, hair, and nails, besides its weight loss benefits.

Red Wine

According to some recent studies, it has been found that drinking red wine under moderation can help in cutting down the extra kilos. Red wine consists of a polyphenol named resveratrol that can aid in losing weight. This very polyphenol can help in converting white fat, the larger cells that store up energy, into beige fat that can deal with obesity. It has also been found that red wine can reduce the risk of a heart attack. In fact, serious problems like Alzheimer's disease and dementia can also be reduced by consuming two glasses of red wine daily. Red wine can also prevent the development of type II diabetes.

Strawberries

Strawberries are filled with fiber, vitamins, polyphenols, zero cholesterol, and zero fat. It is also a great source of magnesium and potassium. You can also get a great deal of vitamin C from strawberries. Consuming one bowl of strawberries every day can help in reducing belly fat. The high fiber content also assists in losing weight. It can help you in staying full that will reduce the chances of overeating or snacking. A hundred grams of strawberries comes with 33 calories only. Strawberries also help in improving the system of digestion and can also readily eliminate toxins from the body. It comes with ellagic acid that can deal with inflammation.

Turmeric

Turmeric is one of the primary spices in every household. It comes with an essential antioxidant called curcumin. It helps in dealing with obesity, disorders related to the stomach, and other health problems. It can help in reducing inflammation that is linked with obesity.

Walnut

Walnuts are rich in healthy fats along with fiber that can aid in losing weight. Walnut can provide you with a great deal of energy as well. It comes with high quantities of PUFAs or polyunsaturated fats that can help in keeping the level of cholesterol under check. Alpha-linolenic acid present in walnuts helps in burning body fat quickly and also promotes proper heart health.

CHAPTER 4: FIRST PHASE OF SIRTDIET - WEIGHT LOSS

The sirtfood diet works in two definite phases that you will need to follow. The whole diet plan lasts for a duration of three weeks. As you complete all the phases of the diet for three weeks, you will need to keep on, including sirtfoods in your daily diet. The more sirtfoods you can include in the diet, the better it will be for you. However, the most important aspect of the sirtdiet is to follow the phases properly. You will need to keep everything under proper check for getting the most out of the diet plan.

The sirtfood diet is all about the food items that have been listed in the previous chapter. Along with all these food items, there are some others as well that you will be able to introduce in all your meals. All the ingredients are quite common and can be found in the market very easily.

The first phase of the sirtfood diet will last for seven days. The aim of this week will be to focus on the restriction of calories. It will be possible to focus on calorie restriction only when you will be able to give up all the carb foods and just concentrate on the green juice. This form of change is necessary for jump-starting the program of weight loss. It is true that this form of change is a sudden drift from any usual form of diet. Thus, the first-week plan has claimed to lose weight by about 3.2 kgs or 7 pounds. The overall intake of calories cannot exceed 1000 and 500 during the first week.

There is a definite branching of calorie intake during the first week. The starting three days of the week will need to be restricted to 1000 calories. Make sure that you do not exceed the calorie count more than that. The diet plant will include essential green juice for three times every day and one meal during the course of the day. You will be able to choose the meals according to you from the recipes that will be mentioned in the latter half of the book. Some sirtfood rich recipes include sirtfood omelet, buckwheat noodles, miso-glazed tofu, and others. After the first three days, the calorie count can be increased only by 500 from the fourth day till the seventh day of the first week. So, you will be able to add one more meal for the day, and you can restrict the essential green juice to two times every day. You will be ending the last four days of the first week with two meals and two glasses of juice.

Green Juice

The green juice plays an important role in the sirtfood diet. Even if you think of not including this juice in your diet, the sirtdiet will not work properly in its absence. It is packed with all the required nutrients and can also act as a great addition to your daily diet. One thing that you will need to keep in mind is that the juice needs to be prepared in a juicer and not in a blender. The green juice can be stored in the refrigerator for about three days, and so it will be better for you to make one large batch for saving time.

Ingredients:

- 2 handfuls of kale
- 30 grams of arugula
- 5 grams parsley

- 5 grams lovage (optional)

- One large stalk of celery with leaves

- One medium-sized green apple

- Half lemon

- Green tea (matcha)

Method:

1. Mix all the greens together (arugula, kale, parsley, and leaves of lovage if you are using them)—Juice all the greens in a juicer. Juicers can differ in their working efficiency while juicing vegetables with leaves. So, you might need to re-juice all the remaining elements in the juicer before you move on to the remaining ingredients. The aim is to make 50 ml of fresh juice from the green elements.

2. After you are done with the greens, juice the green apple and celery.

3. You can put the lemon directly in the juicer after peeling it. But, it will be easier for you if you can squeeze the lemon with your hands into the green juice. By this point in time, you will have about 250 ml of green juice. It can differ depending on the number of ingredients used by you.

4. Pour the green juice in a glass and add matcha green tea in it. Stir the juice properly with the use of a spoon or a fork. After the green tea has dissolved in the juice, give it one more stir and your green juice is ready to drink.

Note: It will be better to use matcha green tea for the first two drinks only as it comes with caffeine. In case you include it in all your drinks, it can readily disturb the sleeping pattern. Also, you can change the consistency of the juice by adding water. Water can be added to change the taste as well.

Day 1	Day 2	Day 3	Day 4	Day 5	Day 6	Day 7
1000 Cals	1000 Cals	1500 Cals	1500 Cals	1500 Cals	1500 Cals	1500 Cals
3 juice and one meal	3 juice and one meal	2 juice and 2 meals	2 juice and 2 meals	2 juice and 2 meals	2 juice and 2 meals	2 juice and 2 meals

Sirtuins

The very first sirtuin was discovered by Dr. Amar Jit

Singh Kar during the 1970s. He names the first sirtuin SIR 2. This is regarded as a gene that comes with the capability of controlling the yeast cell mating. It was in the period between the 1990s when some scientists discovered certain homologous cells to the first sirtuin. Homologous cells are the ones that come with a similar structure as one another. The homologous cells came to be known as sirtuins. From that time, these new genes have been studied in various ways. Sirtuins came to be found in the majority of the organisms which ultimately proved it to be a universal gene. They originated from the ancient times that went through the path of evolution of the organisms. Sirtuins can be found in all the kingdoms and come with a conserved nature of structure. A universal gene is the one that can be found in various organisms. This indicates that the genes were being conserved with the process of evolution of different species.

They come with functions for playing in single or various species that are of universal nature. With the passing time, various studies have been conducted with sirtuins being the primary focus. SIR 2 was the name of the yeast gene that is needed for taking proper care of the cellular functions in yeast. The full form of the gene is silent mating-type information regulation. From all the studies that were being conducted in the condition of in-vitro, it was determined how the genes of SIR 2 implicated the processes of cellular functions in human beings. The roles carried by the gene included apoptosis, aging, inflammation, and transcription. The genes are also capable of resisting stress. In the calorie deficit situations, the genes were also able to control energy efficiency and also resulted in alertness whenever needed.

They act like a family that comes with various proteins

that are capable of controlling cellular health in the bodies of human beings. The proteins give out signals that also help in regulating the metabolic rate. The primary role that was discovered on the part of sirtuins was to control cellular homeostasis. Cellular homeostasis is the process of keeping the cells along with all the functions in proper balance. After conducting various other experiments, it was found that sirtuins are nothing without the presence of NAD+. NAD+ is a coenzyme that can be found universally in the majority of the living cells.

There are certain food items that can activate the sirtuins. Sirtuins that are also called as SIRT can be found in the bodies of human beings. They are total seven in a group ranging from SIRT 1 till SIRT 7. There are various benefits that have been determined by the researchers for all these foods. Such food items come with the capability of mimicking all the benefits related to fasting along with calorie restriction as they can turn the sirtuins active. Various other benefits of sirtuins were discovered with passing time. The benefits include turning on and off certain genes and protecting the body cells from aging. The food items that are capable of activating sirtuins are called sirtfood—the sirtfoods help in turning on the skinny genes.

Sirtuins Present In Human Beings

The total numbers of sirtuins that can be found in human beings are seven. The protein family of SIRT is founded mainly by the yeast gene SIR 2. This protein family tends to play several important roles starting from controlling the chromatin to DNA recombination and gene expression. In the SIRT family, the first three of them, SIRT 1, SIRT 2, and SIRT 3, play the function of deacetylating activity. The other member, SIRT 4, SIRT 5, SIRT 6, and SIRT 7, comes with no or weak deacetylating activity.

Sirtfood Diet

As human beings are warm-blooded in nature, we need proper fuel for performing all the necessary movements. The required fuel is provided by all the foods that we consume daily. Fuel is necessary for keeping up with the functioning of our brain and also for carrying out all the functions normally. The required energy is counted in terms of kilocalories. It has been found that men need 1500 calories, and women need 1200 calories minimum for performing all the necessary functions. All those who suffer from obesity and are very much tensed about losing the extra kilos think that it is the calories only that plays a role in regulating body weight. But, in actual, it depends on each and everything that we consume.

SIRT 1 that is present in the human cells helps in extending the lifespan and also participates in inducing the new formation of mitochondria in the body cells. Besides all these, it also helps in improving the oxidative type of metabolism that is necessary for supporting weight loss along with maintenance of the same. Sirtfoods, as provided in the sirtdiet, turns on the sirtuin proteins that participate in shedding the extra fat in the body. Thus, you can lose weight within just one week during the first phase of the diet. As the intake of calories is restricted to 1000 during the first three days of the first phase, you will be losing the extra kilos while you will be getting all the energy that is being provided by the body. The body provides all the energy by burning down stored fat and turns it into glycogen.

The people who are the masterminds behind the creation of sirtfoods claimed that the food items in the diet can activate all those mechanisms that are actually controlled by the sirt genes or skinny genes. The skinny gene is present in the human body that can help in burning down fat. Thus, it ultimately leads to weight loss. Sirtfood diet can sound very appealing in nature as it consists of all those food items that we all love. The diet emphasizes on food items such as berries, kale, chocolate, coffee, red wine, olive oil, turmeric, and others that have already been discussed in the previous chapter. All the food items that are included in this diet are mainly plant-based, which can help in activating the sirtuins by stimulating all the proteins that are encoded for the gene of SIRT 1. As you restrict your daily calorie intake, it can show a positive impact on your life, such as improving your lifespan. Thus, sirtfoods plays the primary role by turning on the pathways that are sirt-mediated and also by turning on the activity of burning fat. It can also help in supercharging weight loss and staving off various diseases.

CHAPTER 5: SECOND PHASE OF SIRTDIET - MAINTENANCE

The second phase of the sirtfood diet is the last phase of the whole diet. It will be lasting for a period of two weeks. During this phase, you will need to maintain the routine by which you have been consuming food in the first phase of the sirtdiet. All that you will need to do is to keep a check on the calorie count so that the weight loss can be steady. The diet that you will be following will look somewhat like this: one green juice and three meals of sirtfoods in a day. You will be able to choose the recipes that you would like, that are focused mainly on sirtfoods.

The second phase of the sirtdiet is known as the maintenance stage. All the real magic lies in this phase, in spite of the fact that you will be losing about 3 kgs in the first phase. This stage is more about maintaining that you have lost during the first phase. The maintenance stage might turn out to be a bit tough as there is no definite restriction on calorie intake and so you might regain all the weight that you have lost.

As you are specific about the type of food that you will be consuming and also the nutritional value that they possess, the most beneficial thing is not to consider what passes through the food pipe to the stomach. It is more about the way in which your body is capable of absorbing all the nutrients and makes the best use of them. If you add nice and colored veggies and fruits in the diet, there is no doubt that it will be adding more nutrients in all the meals. But, you will also need to pay attention to the absorption of the nutrients by the body. The ability of the body to absorb the necessary nutrients from the meals that are termed as bioavailability is equally important as the nutrient content of the foods that we consume.

There are various food items that can be combined with others for assisting the body in nutrient absorption. It is believed that when two types of foods are combined with each other, they can have more essential effects on the human body in comparison to consuming them all alone. This is termed as food synergy. This helps in explaining why we tend to develop a definite taste for the consumption of certain food items together. It can also help in describing the type of interaction that exists between the food items for providing benefits to your health and body system. So, for improving the bioavailability of the nutrients in the meals, you will need to take care of the relationship of nutrient synergy as you decide the meal menus. Some examples of food combinations are red pepper and quinoa, avocado and tomato, turmeric and black pepper, and so on.

Tips For Sticking To Your Diet Plan

As you eat healthily and follow a proper diet plan, you can easily cut off the extra pounds from your body. It will also allow you to improve the levels of your energy. In fact, following a diet plan like sirtfood diet can help in improving your mood and can also lower the risk of developing chronic diseases. But, in spite of all these benefits, sticking to your diet might turn out to be challenging. Here are certain ways by which you can stick to your diet plan.

Starting With Expectations That Are Real

Being on a nutritious diet comes along with various benefits along with potential loss of body weight. But, it is also very important to set up expectations that are realistic by nature. For instance, if you start pressurizing yourself for losing your body weight very quickly, the whole plan of achieving better health might actually backfire. In the case of sirtdiet, you will be able to lose about 3 kgs in the first phase. If you are thinking of losing about 5 – 6 kgs in one week, you will never be able to stick to the diet plan. As you set an achievable and realistic goal, it will prevent you from losing all the motivation and can also help you in losing weight consistently.

Thinking About All Those Things That Can Motivate You

If you can remember or make yourself aware of the fact why you are opting for weight loss and healthy eating choices, it can help you a lot in being on the course. If you want, you can also make a list of various reasons why you are willing to turn to a healthy diet plan. You will need to keep this reason list handy so that you can refer to the same whenever you need a reminder.

Keeping Food Items Out Of Reach That Is Not Included In The Plan

It will be difficult for you to eat healthy and stick to the diet plan if you remain surrounded by unhealthy foods. In case other members of the family want to consume them, you can try to keep them in any hidden spot in place of keeping it on the shelves or countertop. The very famous saying, out of your sight and out of your mind, can be applied here. You can try keeping all those foods items that are not included in the diet plan out of your hands, or you can even someone else to hide them for you. This will help in readily preventing you from munching on unhealthy foods that can aid in losing weight. It has been found that displaying unhealthy foods or food items that are not included in the plan can lead to obesity or even more consumption of junk foods.

Not Having All Or Nothing Kind Of Approach

One of the major hurdles in the pathway to achieve a healthy lifestyle and diet is thinking black and white. For example, you are at a party with various unhealthy food items around you. You will think that the day is completely ruined and you will get indulged in eating those unhealthy foods. This should not be the case. In place of thinking that the day is completely ruined, try opting for the healthy and unprocessed food items at the party. If possible, try to opt for high protein foods. This will be helping you in feeling full, along with a feeling of satisfaction rather than feeling frustrated and stuffed. Certain choices that are off the plan can make very small differences in the long term, as long as you can balance all of them with foods of healthy nature.

Carrying Healthy Snacks

It might turn out to be a daunting task to stick to your healthy diet plan when you are not at home for a long period. When you feel hungry as you are on the go, it can result in grabbing anything that is available in front of you. In the majority of the cases, it is processed food that cannot really make you feel full. They are not fit for the long term. You can carry healthy protein snacks such as protein bar so that you can keep a check on your appetite before you opt for a full meal. Some other examples of portable snacks are peanuts, almonds, protein shakes, etc. You can also opt for a mini cooler for carrying cheese, boiled eggs, and yogurt.

Exercising And Changing The Diet At Same Point

You must have heard that you should not opt for changing many things at a time when you are thinking of improving the quality of your health. In actuality, this is a great piece of advice. However, various research depicted that when someone opts for physical as well as dietary changes at the same point of time, the end results can actually reinforce one another. In a research with 200 people, all those who opted for a healthy diet and physical activity at the same time found the whole thing much easier to maintain all the behaviors in comparison to all those who opted for exercise or diet alone. As you begin exercising and opting for a healthy diet simultaneously, it can easily improve the overall chances of succeeding in a healthy lifestyle.

Having A Game Plan Before Consuming Food

Giving in your all for maintaining a healthy diet while also eating out might turn out to be very challenging in nature. However, there are certain ways to make the whole game easier. For example, you can opt for checking out the menu before you go out to a place or having water before the meal. It is always a great idea to have a proper strategy in your mind before you opt for going out to a restaurant instead of just feeling overwhelmed after you reach there.

Do Not Allow Your Travelling Schedule To Derail You

No matter if you are traveling for pleasure or business, staying outside your regular territory can actually make it a bit tough to stay by a healthy diet plan. There are certain tips that you can follow for sticking to your diet plan.

- Try to do your research about the supermarkets and restaurants of the place where you are heading to. Checking these things out ahead of time can help in aiding your diet plan.

- Try to carry some healthy food items with you that do not get spoiled very easily.

- Try to challenge yourself for being on track for the majority of the trip.

Practicing Mindful Eating

When you opt for mindful eating, it will make it a lot easier for you to maintain your diet plan and stay healthy. Take as much time as you want to enjoy your food. Try to appreciate the ability of the food items to nourish your health. This will easily increase the chances of being successful on the journey to a healthy lifestyle, along with lasting changes in your behavior. In a study of five months, obese and overweight women who opted for mindful eating improved their food relationships significantly. Also, if you opt for mindful eating, you can easily deal with your habit of binge eating.

Tracking And Monitoring The Progress

Logging the food items that you consume daily in a diary, app, or online food tracker can help a lot in sticking to a healthy diet. It will also help you in your venture of losing weight. You can also opt for measuring your progress of exercising as it can provide you with all the motivation that you need for going on. As you can see the progress in your diary or tracker, it will motivate you and strengthen your mindset for being on the path.

Getting A Partner For Joining You

Sticking to an exercise plan along with healthy eating might turn out to be a tough game if you opt for doing it on your own, all alone. When you have an exercise or diet buddy, it can help you a lot in sticking to the plan. It can work the best of the partner is your spouse or best friend. You will be able to feel motivated when you have someone by your side who is on the same journey as you. Also, in case you feel demotivated, the other partner can help in keeping up the spirit.

Realizing That It Will Take Time For Changing The Habits

There is nothing to lose all your courage if it takes a long time to adapt to the new habits and routines. It will obviously take some time to change all that you have been doing for a long time. Try to bring about the changes slowly and do not just rush for it. Eventually, exercising and eating healthy will turn out to be automatic.

Figuring Out What Will Work Out The Best

No one can find a perfect way that will work out for all. It is very important to figure out a way of exercising and eating that you can actually enjoy.

Breaking your old habits and improving the diet is not an easy game. But, all these strategies can help in sticking to the diet plans and for assisting in weight loss. Just determine a target and work towards it slowly instead of just jumping right to the conclusion.

CHAPTER 6: AFTER THE DIET

After you are done with the diet, you can repeat the phases again according to your target of losing weight. Even when you achieve the target, the diet creators suggest that adopting various types of sirtfoods in your daily meals can help a lot. This is because the diet has been designed in a way that can be treated as an alternate way of living. This indicates that after you are done with the three-week diet, you can continue having the same meals along with the green juice. Besides all these, you can opt for certain other things as well for reaping most of the benefits of the diet.

- **Resume the routines of workout:** As you will be limiting your calorie consumption during the initial days of the diet, it is always recommended to lessen or just stop exercising until the body gets accustomed to the brand new conditions. No person can be like the other. So, the best way of determining when you can again start with your old routine of workout is by paying attention to the body. For being on the safe side, the majority of the diet followers opt for resuming the regular workout routine after they are done with the second phase of the sirtdiet. By that point in time, you will be able to analyze your levels of energy, and you will also be able to complete tougher sets of your exercise.

- **Try out protein powder with sirtfood smoothies:** In case you think of exercising again, you will need to add smoothies to the diet that contains protein powder along with sirtfoods. This will help in dealing with muscle soreness and will also help in keeping up your energy levels after exercising. Recipes for tasty smoothies will be provided at the end of the book. If you are sure about your kitchen skills, you can experiments with sirtfoods for finding out the perfect smoothie.

- **Inviting your friends and family for the diet:** One of the perfect ways of maintaining a healthy diet is by getting others around you opt for the diet as well. It has been found that having the perfect kind of company can actually have a great influence on your routine. You can show your family and friends the various benefits of the diet so that they also opt for the same.

You can consider adapting to the principles of this diet as a normal part of your daily life. It is up to you whether you want to add sirtfoods in your daily diet or not.

Turning The Diet In Your Daily Lifestyle

As you practice the diet with exercising, it is tough to consume protein right after half an hour of finishing the workout. Protein helps in fixing the muscles after a session of exercise, helps in recuperation, and also lessens irritation. There are various protein–rich sirt smoothies that you can opt for, such as a blueberry smoothie with some protein powder in it. The sirtdiet is actually a great way of changing the patterns of your diet, lose weight, and get the feeling of being advantageous. You will need to keep a check on the nourishments that are perfect for you to eat and also which plan will suit you the best.

You can include supplements such as vitamin B6 and B12, iron, calcium, vitamin B9, vitamin E, and vitamin C.

CHAPTER 7: SIRTFOOD DIET AND WORKOUT

Sirtdiet can be regarded as a way of life rather than one single time diet plan. For the majority of us, it might actually be a tough job to lose weight or just retain a normal body weight. But, with the help of sirtdiet, all those people who are struggling with weight loss can lose weight easily. However, is it possible to combine exercising with a sirtfood diet, or do we need to keep our workout routines out of the way?

With about 700 million adults who are suffering from obesity all over the world, it is essential to look out for a healthy way of eating and regimes of exercising that are actually doable. Something is needed that will not be depriving you of enjoying your life and will not need you to keep on exercising all throughout the week. All these things can be done single-handedly by the sirtfood diet. The primary idea is that some food items will be activating the skinny gene, which is generally turned on with the help of exercising and fasting. During the first and second phases of the diet, it will be good for you if you can stop exercising or reduce the intensity of the same. This is because sirtdiet is mainly about restricting your calorie intake. As you reduce your physical activities, it will be easier for the body to adapt to the fewer amount of calories.

You will need to listen to the body. In case you are feeling low in energy or if you feel fatigued, stop working out for a few days. Dedicate that time in remaining focused on the sirtdiet principles for a healthy life.

Exercising After The Diet

It is completely okay to get back to your workout routine after you are done with both the phases of the diet. But, make sure that you include enough protein in your daily diet for aiding in muscle recovery. The best part about sirtdiet is that there is no risk of losing your muscles. It will be reducing the fat content only, and so even the athletes can opt for a sirtfood diet. You will need to be kind to yourself during the initial weeks as your body adapts to the changes routine. If you have the habit of exercising moderately all throughout the year, you can exercise at the time of diet as well. It will depend on you, how far you will be able to push yourself for bringing about the required change in your life. Just manage your fitness regime according to your diet regime.

Importance Of Exercising

Exercising involves all those movements that can allow your body to burn out calories and make muscles work. You can opt for various types of physical exercises such as running, walking, jogging, swimming, dancing, and so on. As you start being active, it can showcase various benefits over your health, both mental and physical. In fact, coupling exercises with a sirtfood diet can help in shedding extra pounds and obviously moderate exercising.

Can Give You A Happy Feeling

Exercise can help in uplifting your mood. It can also deal with depression, stress, and anxiety. As you start with sirtfood diet, your body will enter a state of shock during the first few days as you will be restricting the calories suddenly. Moderate exercising can help in dealing with stress of this kind. Exercising can bring about certain changes in the brain that can regulate anxiety and stress. In fact, it can also help in improving the sensitivity of the brain for hormones such as norepinephrine and serotonin that helps in relieving depression.

Also, exercising can improve the production of the hormone endorphins that deals with positive feelings and also help in dealing with pain. Exercise has shown positive effects on people who suffer from anxiety. With moderate exercising, you will be able to be aware of your mental state. You can also opt for distractions for coping up with fears. It does not matter how intensively you exercise. You will be able to benefit even from moderate exercise. As you cut down calories during the first phase of the diet, you are most likely to develop a disturbing mood. Exercise can play a deep role in regulating your mood. In fact, people who opt for exercising along with sirtdiet showed better results in comparison to all those who opted for the diet alone.

Exercising And Weight Loss

The main aim of sirtdiet is to cut off the extra pounds from your body. As you stay inactive or get indulged in very less physical activities, it can result in obesity and weight gain. For understanding the overall effect of exercising on the reduction of weight, you will need to have a clear understanding of the relationship between energy expenditure and exercise. The human body is capable of spending energy in three definite ways: exercising, food digestion, and maintenance of body functions such as breathing and heartbeat. As you start with the diet, the calorie intake will be reduced, and that will be lowering the rate of metabolism. This might result in delaying the loss of weight. On the other hand, exercising along with your diet plan can improve the metabolic rate that will help in burning down more calories. Thus, you will be able to lose more weight without any effect on your muscle mass.

It has been found that the combination of aerobic exercise and resistance training can improve the loss of fat and can also help in the maintenance of muscle mass. So, make sure that you opt for moderate exercising after you are done with the two phases of the diet.

Exercising Is Beneficial For The Bones And Muscles

Exercise can play a beneficial role in maintaining and building strong bones and muscles. Physical type of activity such as weight lifting can help in building muscles when it is coupled with proper intake of protein. This is mainly because exercise helps in releasing certain hormones that can promote the capability of the muscles for absorbing amino acids. This ultimately helps in growing and reducing the breakdown. With growing age, people tend to lose their muscle mass along with their function. This can result in disabilities and injuries. It is essential to opt for physical activities daily for retaining the mass of the muscles at the time of following a diet. It can help in maintaining your strength with age.

Exercising can help in improving the density of the

bones that can help a lot in preventing osteoporosis at a later stage in life. Exercises that involve high impacts such as running or gymnastics or sports such as basketball and soccer have shown to improve bone density at a higher rate in comparison to non-impact activities such as cycling and swimming.

Improvement Of Energy Levels

Exercise comes with the great power of boosting your energy level. In case you are suffering from any sort of medical condition, it can help in improving your energy in that case as well. In sirtdiet, energy is provided by the body by burning down body fat. When you couple it with proper exercise, you can improve the benefits of the same. Exercising can help in boosting the energy levels of all those people who suffer from CFS or chronic fatigue syndrome. It is possible to treat other illnesses like AIDS and cancer with the help of proper exercise and diet.

Exercise Can Reduce Chronic Diseases

When there is a lack of physical activity, it can lead to chronic diseases. With the help of regular exercise, it can help in improving sensitivity to insulin, body composition, and also cardiovascular fitness. It can also help in maintaining blood pressure along with the levels of body fat. In fact, lack of physical exercise, even for a short period, can result in the development of body fat and can also increase the overall risk of developing diabetes of type 2. Physical exercise is necessary with proper diet for reducing belly fat percentage.

Improves Skin Health

The quality of the skin can get affected by a high

amount of oxidative stress on the body. Oxidative stress takes place when the antioxidant defenses of the body are unable to mend the damage that is caused to the cells by the free radicals. This can result in damaging the internal structures and can also lead to deterioration of the skin quality. It is true that exhaustive and intense physical activity can result in oxidative damage; moderate exercising daily can improve the production of antioxidants naturally. This can help in protecting the skin cells. Similarly, exercising can help in stimulating the flow of blood and can also induce adaptations of the skin cells that contribute to delaying the occurrence of skin aging.

Improve Brain Memory And Health

It has been found that the functioning of the brain can be improved with the help of regular exercise. It can also help in protecting your memory and skills of thinking. For beginning with it, it can help in improving the heart rate that can promote a better flow of blood along with oxygen to the brain. In fact, the production of hormones can be simulated that can directly help in enhancing the overall growth of the brain cells. Regular exercise with a proper diet is more important for older adults as with the increased rate of inflammation and oxidative stress; it can also lead to changes in the structure of the brain along with its functioning.

Exercise Can Improve The Quality Of Sleep

Regular exercise with a balanced diet can help in relaxing and also sound sleep. While talking about sleep quality, the depletion of energy that takes place at the time of sirtdiet helps in stimulating the recuperative processes at the time of sleep. This whole thing gets boosted when the diet is coupled with moderate exercise. Moreover, as you exercise, it also increases the temperature of the body that can also improve the quality of your sleep. In elderly people, the problem of sleep disorders tends to be readily available. Exercising can help in dealing with sleep disorders as well. You can be completely flexible regarding the type of exercise that you want to choose. It has been found that aerobic exercise, coupled with resistance training, can improve sleep quality more in comparison to opting for any one of them.

Exercise Can Help In Reducing Pain

Chronic pain might turn out to be debilitating. But, with the help of exercise, you can deal with it very easily. Exercising helps in toning the muscles that remain inactive, and this, in turn, results in the reduction of pain. You will be able to improve your level of pain tolerance and also decrease the perception of pain with the help of daily exercise.

Athletes can opt for sirtdiet along with regular exercising as there is no need to be inactive and it does not even affect the muscle mass. You will be able to boost up the functioning of your immune system as well.

CHAPTER 8: COSTS

No matter what type of diet you opt for, it will always come with a definite cost. The same goes for the sirtfood diet as well. But, unlike other diets, it is quite economical in nature and will not be costing you much after the first few initial expenses. You will need to get a juicer for preparing the green juice along with certain expensive items that will be raising the initial costs a bit. However, once you have started with the diet, it will not cost you much. The main reason behind this is that you will be consuming only one or two meals a day according to your choice.

The best part about sirtdiet is that you are not needed to be an excellent athlete or a sportsperson for reaping all the benefits of this wonderful diet. There is no requirement of excessive calorie restriction. It will not be consuming much of your time and is inexpensive as well. In fact, the majority of the food items that are included in the diet can be found easily in the market. So, it can be said that sirtdiet is an economical way of shedding the extra pounds.

Shopping At The Perimeter

In most of the cases, healthy and fresh protein sources are placed at the perimeter of the local stores. The internal aisles contain other healthy food items such as beans, canned nuts, and so on, along with unhealthy food items such as soda, candy, chips, and others. You will need to make sure that you fill your shopping cart with the perimeter items before moving for the internal aisles. Also, you will need to ensure that you fill your basket with various types of vegetables along with fruits. All the fruits and vegetables that are included in the diet are readily available. In case you want to add some colors to your diet, you can do that. That includes opting for colorful varieties such as red peppers, greens, berries, turmeric, sweet potatoes, etc.

Colorful food items are loaded with important plant compounds that are essential for the body. It is always recommended to be prepared right before you start cooking to ensure that your kitchen is filled with all the important items. In this way, you will also be able to track your wellness goals. You can buy the grocery items that can you can store in your pantry for use at any time when you want.

It is always very tempting to look out for the fad diets that can help in cutting down the calories extensively. But, they should not be opted for if you are very much concerned about weight loss for the long term. It is always of great priority whenever we discuss opting for a particular method of losing weight that is both sustainable and healthy. You can opt for clean eating to serve this purpose. You will be dealing with a diet plan that you can follow for your entire life where there is no need for any unhealthy tactics for losing weight. Also, you will not need to deprive your own self of all your cravings. It is very easy, just like keeping away processed foods and depending on the whole food items for the improvement of your health in various ways.

It has been found that combining new food items with

all your clean foods can help you in sticking to the diet. With this method, you will be able to follow a lifestyle while also getting the chance to expand your food palate. You can try out various types of veggies and spices for making your diet plan interesting. The majority of the people try to opt for food items that are low in overall fat count, specifically all the dressings that are used for preparing the meals. There are certain types of dressings that come with preservatives and additives. So, it will be better for you to prepare your own food dressings. It will be tastier than the preserved ones and will also help in cutting down a lot of your expenses. Try to opt for whole food items such as unsweetened food items, full-fat yogurt, and so on.

CHAPTER 9: SIDE EFFECT AND CONTRADICTIONS

Sirtfood diet can readily help in losing a great amount of weight during the first phase of the diet as it is all about restricting the calorie intake. But, all of this is only for a short period. What is going to happen if you stop following the diet after the second phase? A definite question will always remain in the air regarding the overall effectiveness of the sirtfood diet. Many people are still very doubtful whether this diet plan is only a silly diet trend. If that is the case, does the diet have any kind of positive side?

In the first place, the primary complaint of the majority of people who opted for the sirtfood diet is regarding the restrictive nature of the diet. Other weight-loss diets, such as the keto diet, also aim to lose weight. But, such diets also take care of providing the body with a balanced sort of nutrient supply. However, the sirtfood diet focuses primarily on the intake of calories. Certain groups of food items that are regarded as being the major ones are also kept out of the diet list. It also involves downsizing the portions to an excessive level. It is more likely to lose a certain amount of lean protein at the early stage from the poultry, beef, legumes, and other food items. But, you will be allowed to introduce olive oil and walnuts which are taken as the sources of sirtuins. However, the daily calorie count for the starting two weeks is actually less than 50% of the overall requirement of an average individual. Other important nutrients that are needed for a healthy body such as calcium and iron are also absent in the sirtfood diet.

The fact about the sirtuins that it can result in weight loss is still an unclear aspect, to begin with. Until now, no form of research has been conducted for determining the link between sirtuin–rich food items and weight loss. It is regarded that sustaining on the green juice for a long time while also cutting down sugar from the food items can result in weight loss for any person. In fact, some major groups of food items are kept out of the list so that it can aid in weight loss. It is actually a very natural thing that consuming fewer calories while also staying hydrated can help in shedding all the unnecessary pounds. Nothing is there that can make it look great, and it actually makes sense.

So, it turns out to be a tricky task to determine whether the change in weight is actually a result of following the sirtdiet during the two phases and is dependent on the diet that is low in calories or is the result of the power of the involved food items that activates the sirtuins for burning the unnecessary fat. In fact, when the related food items are not included in the diet, anyone can lose weight if they follow a diet that comes with restrictive calorie consumption. In case you are very sure that you are shedding some extra kilos when you follow the diet, it might actually be the water weight that is being shed. You will be gaining back all those extra kilos right after you get back to your normal diet plan that you have following before the sirtdiet that comes with more consumption of calories.

It has been found that the quick weight loss that can be achieved with sirtdiet can actually slow down the metabolic rate of the body as the body will be adapting its functions to a lowered calorie consumption process. In the second place, sirtfood diet is nothing special or different than the other forms of diets that can have contradictions or side effects. It is true that sirtdiet will not be doing much harm to the body as it is for a very short term. But, it can still result in various types of issues in case you have the habit of eating a lot during the course of the day. The issues can include distorted mental focus, fatigue, nausea, headache, and others. But, you can also achieve something positive from the diet. Sirtdiet can readily help in improving the condition of your heart health. The main reason behind this is the polyphenols that can be found in abundance in food items that are included for sirtdiet.

The end result of the diet might be that the weight you have just lost after sustaining to all the phases might not last long because of the restrictive nature of the diet. In case you have any form of a complicated relationship with food consumption habits, it will be better for you if you can skip the diet. This is mainly because you might end up with overeating after the diet gets over, which can result in harmful effects for the body.

CHAPTER 10: QUESTIONS AND ANSWERS

As sirtdiet is a new topic in the world of diet, there are various questions that are being asked by all those people who are willing to opt for it. Well, sirtdiet is a simple thing, and it is not much complicated. Let's have a look at some of the most widely asked questions along with the answers of the same.

Can I Exercise During The First Phase Of The Diet?

Normal exercise is the best thing that can be done for the improvement of your health. Opting for mild exercise can help in improving the loss of weight along with various medical advantages during the first phase of the sirtfood diet. In case you are having doubt of any kind, it is always recommended to proceed with the regular degree of physical movement and exercises all throughout the first week of the diet. It is always better to be within the boundary of your own safe place. Exceptional or delayed exercising can add extra weight to the body. All that you will need to do is to tune in to the level of your body. There is no need to push yourself for excessive exercising during the first phase of the diet. Just leave it upon the sirtfoods for accomplishing all the tough work.

Can I Opt For Sirtdiet If I Am Underweight Or Excessively Thin?

It is not recommended to opt for a sirtfood diet if a person is underweight. An easy way of checking whether you have a normal weight or underweight is by computing your record of weight or BMI. You can check your BMI according to the height and weight of your body on various online calculators. In case the BMI is 18.5 or even less than that, it is not recommended to opt for the diet. If your BMI is between 18.5 and 21, it is actually an alarming sign as following the diet can result in lowering the BMI underneath the mark of 18.5. Although several people have the urge to be super-thin, it can have various contradictions for the body. It includes adding up to a resistant nature of the framework, increased risk of developing osteoporosis, issues with fruitfulness, and others.

It is not at all recommended to start with the diet if a person is underweight, but in case you want to add some sirtfoods to your daily diet, you can do that. If you have the BMI range of 20 – 25, there is nothing that can prevent you from opting for the diet.

Can I Stop Following The Diet After Achieving The Target Body Weight?

Firstly, congratulations on achieving your target body weight. You must have achieved the target weight, but the journey will not be ending right now while it is not suggested to opt for any more calorie restriction, the diet that you will be following needs to have a sufficient number of sirtfoods. There is no harm in including sirtfoods in your daily diet. The best thing about sirtfoods is that they are more of a lifestyle than a diet. If you try to stop the diet right now, it might result in gaining back the lost weight once again. So, it is always suggested to include certain sirtfoods in your daily diet for keeping up with healthy body weight.

Can I Stop Drinking The Green Juice After Completing The Second Phase Of The Diet?

Green juice is the core of the sirtfood diet. No other food item can provide you with the effectiveness of green juice. The green juice can provide you with supplements that can actuate the sirtuins for boosting weight loss. But, it depends completely on you whether you want to continue with the green juice or just discard the same from your daily diet. In case you do not like the taste of the juice, you can experiment with the taste by adding your favorite items in it.

Can I Follow The Sirtdiet While Taking Medicinal Drugs?

The sirtdiet is all about altering the metabolic rate and

targeting weight loss. So, there are chances that it can play with the effects of the medicines that are prescribed by your physician. There are certain types of drugs that are not at all suitable for the state of fasting. In case you can feel any kind of adverse effects of the medicines during the first phase of the diet, it is always suggested to stop with the diet. Consult your physician in the first place if you are facing certain odds with the diet and medicines.

Can I Follow The Diet At The Time Of Pregnancy?

Sirtfood diet can be included in your daily diet, no matter what the case is. It comes with a nourishing effect on your wellbeing and health. But, as a sirtfood diet does not include certain nutrients and food groups in the diet, it can result in nutrient deficiency at the time of pregnancy. You will need to check about the same with your doctor first before starting with the diet. Also, you will need to keep red wine out of the list because of the alcoholic substances present in it. You cannot have stimulating food items such as espresso, cocoa, or green tea because of the caffeine content.

How Frequently Can I Opt For The Phases Of The Diet?

The first phase can opt at any time when you feel that you require some loss of body weight, or you need to cut down some excess pounds. But, you will need to keep a considerable gap in between before opting for the first phase again. The second phase can be carried out whenever you like as this stage is more like a lifestyle.

CHAPTER 11: RECIPES

This chapter is all about the various types of recipes that you can include in your sirtfood diet. Sirtdiet is mainly based on the first phase. So, you can arrange the recipes according to your choice in a 7-day meal plan that works the best for you.

It will be easier for you to alter the eating habits along with the habits of grocery shopping when you follow a definite meal plan. It will also be helping you to discard all those food items that are unhealthy and preserved from the chart of your diet plan. You will be able to save a lot of your time by preparing a proper meal plan first by incorporating only certain limited food items in your grocery list. It will help you to make new meals with the various types of recipes. In fact, you will also get the opportunity to store the leftover food in the refrigerator for use at a later time. You will get the chance to satisfy the members of your family by preparing the favorite recipes, and all of this can be achieved by preparing a meal plan.

The best part about a meal plan is that you will be able to cut down the wastage of food. You will be able to enjoy a happy life with your family. You will be capable of achieving the perfect body weight by focusing on nutritional and well-balanced meals per day. It will be allowing you to maintain the needed level of nutrition by the body with the right meal plan. You can try out a variety of options for healthy salads and soups by keeping junk foods out of the list. Also, homemade meals that are prepared with ingredients low in calories can help in reducing the risk of various chronic diseases. It might happen that you don't get enough time to prepare timely meals every day. In that case, preparing a meal plan and refrigerating the food can help in maintaining your exact routine of meals. In this way, you will be able to free yourself from the burden of cooking as you return home from work after a long and tiring day.

A proper meal plan can help in handling your stress level as you will need less amount of time along with money for preparing the same. So, let's have a look at some of the sirtdiet recipes that can help in setting your meal plan easily.

Cherry And Strawberry Smoothie

Total Prep & Cooking Time: 5 minutes

Yields: 5 Servings

Nutrition Facts: Calories: 95 | Protein: 2g | Fat: 2g | Carbs: 22.3g | Fiber: 7g

Ingredients:

- 2 cups frozen or fresh strawberries
- 2 cups frozen or fresh sweet cherries
- One cup of water
- One large orange (properly peeled with separated wedges)
- One large banana
- One tbsp. of chia seeds
- Agave nectar or honey (optional)

Method:

1. Use an electric blender for combining all the ingredients. You will need to add the ingredients in the blender in the order as they are enlisted. As the normal rule, you will need to add the frozen ingredients at the last and the liquid first. The other ingredients will go in between the two. Blend the smoothie until smooth.

2. In case you want to enjoy the smoothie a bit sweet, you can add agave nectar or honey to the smoothie after blending. Blend it once more for a few seconds, and you are good to go.

Notes:

- If you want to have the smoothie chilled, it will be better to use frozen cherries and strawberries.

- The strawberries and cherries can be stored in the refrigerator after pitting. You will be able to enjoy the goodness of smoothies during the winters as well.

- You will be able to enjoy the smoothie all throughout the year, as you can use both frozen and fresh strawberries along with cherries for the smoothie.

- Cherries and strawberries are rich in antioxidants. It can help in lowering the risk of various types of diseases like heart diseases, blood sugar, diabetes, and so on. The fruits used for this smoothie are rich in fiber as well that important for weight management after reducing the intake of calories.

Mango Ginger Kale Smoothie

Total Prep & Cooking Time: 4 minutes

Yields: 3 Servings

Nutrition Facts: Calories: 119 | Protein: 2.4g | Fat: 0.9g | Carbs: 26.8g | Fiber: 4g

Ingredients:

One cup of each:

- Frozen ripe mango cubes
- Frozen ripe peaches
- Two cups of kale (frozen or fresh)
- One tbsp. of minced ginger
- One cup ice
- Two limes or lemons (juiced)
- Two cups of water

- One tbsp. of maple syrup (optional)

Method:

1. Start by adding ice to the blender. Crush the ice.

2. Add mango cubes, peaches, kale, lemon juice, ginger, and one cup water to the blender. The total amount of water that you will need to add will depend on the number of frozen items.

3. Blend the ingredients until properly smooth. You can add water in between if needed or for altering the consistency. Scrape the sides of the blender in between.

4. After you are done with blending the ingredients, taste it and add seasonings if needed according to your taste. You can use more fruits or maple syrup if the mixture is too tart. In case you want

to add zing to the smoothie, add minced ginger. For adding acidity to the smoothie, you can add more juice of a lemon. For making the smoothie colder or thicker, add more amount of ice. You can blend the smoothie as needed.

5. Serve immediately after you are done with blending. The leftover smoothie can be stored in the refrigerator for later use for one day.

Notes:

- This smoothie is loaded with greens and is tart as well.

- In case you are looking out for a smoothie that is not too sweet creamy, this is a perfect choice.

- You can adjust the flavors according to your taste.

Mixed Berry Summer Smoothie

Total Prep & Cooking Time: 5 minutes

Yields: 2 Servings

Nutrition Facts: Calories: 222 | Protein: 5g | Fat: 0.9g | Carbs: 51g | Fiber: 3g

Ingredients:

- Two cups of apple juice
- One large banana (sliced)
- One cup of Greek yogurt
- Two cups of mixed berries (frozen)
- One tbsp. of honey (optional)
- Mint springs and fresh berries (optional; for garnishing)

Method:

1. Take a blender and add banana, apple juice, yogurt, and berries. Blend the ingredients until smooth. In case the smoothie is a bit thick, you can add a bit more liquid (about half a cup).

2. Taste the smoothie and add honey to it if you want. Divide the smoothie into two glasses and top it with mint springs and fresh berries.

Notes:

- You can also use skim milk, almond milk, coconut milk, or some other liquid in place of apple juice.

- You can have this smoothie as a great start to your day or also as a mid-day snack.

- It can mend your hunger and can also make you feel refreshed.

- It is rich in protein because of the Greek yogurt.

Green Grape Smoothie

Total Prep & Cooking Time: 7 minutes

Yields: 2 servings

Nutrition Facts: Calories: 298 | Carbs: 19g | Protein: 0.75g | Fat: 0.18g | Fiber: 0.8g

Ingredients:

- One cup seedless grapes (green)
- One cup of almond milk (sweetened)
- Two tsps. honey
- One medium cucumber (peeled and sliced thinly)
- Two medium-sized celery stalks along with leaves

Method:

1. Take a blender and add all the ingredients one by one. Make sure that you start with the almond milk first and then add the rest of the ingredients. Turn on the blender and blend the ingredients until the smoothie turns smooth and frothy.

2. Divide the smoothie into two glasses and serve immediately.

Note: The leftover smoothie can be stored in the freezer for later consumption.

Orange and Celery Juice

Total Prep & Cooking Time: 25 minutes

Yields: 4 servings

Nutrition Facts: Calories: 112 | Carbs: 27g | Protein: 2.5g | Fat: 0.9g | Fiber: 6.3g

Ingredients:

- Six medium–sized carrots (properly peeled and chopped into cubes)
- Four celery sticks (properly peeled and chopped)
- 700 ml of fresh orange juice

For garnishing:

- Two sticks of celery, properly peeled and cut into halves
- Celery leaves

Method:

1. Take a blender or food processor and add celery, carrots, and orange juice to it. Blend the ingredients until properly smooth. Make sure that you check the consistency of the smoothie in between and add orange juice according to your need. Blend the mixture once again.

2. Allow the smoothie to remain in the blender for some time. Let the smoothie chill.

3. After the smoothie is chilled according to your desired level, pour the smoothie out of the blender.

4. Divide the smoothie into four tall glasses. Add sticks of celery from the top and garnish with celery leaves.

Notes:

• Celery can help a lot in losing weight. It comes along with dietary fibers that can help in boosting the overall process related to digestion. One large celery stalk contains about ten calories only. Food items that are low in calorie count are generally preferred the most when it comes to the shedding of extra pounds. Along with that, celery comes with a great percentage of water and electrolytes that can help in preventing dehydration.

- Orange also comes with a low-calorie count. So, celery and orange together can help a lot in losing all the excess body weight.

Kale Blackcurrant Smoothie

Total Prep & Cooking Time: 10 minutes

Yields: 4 Servings

Nutrition Facts: Calories: 201 | Protein: 2.5g | Fat: 11.3g | Carbs: 20g | Fiber: 10g

Ingredients:

Two tbsps. of each:

- Wheatgrass
- Honey
- One large avocado (sliced)
- 500 ml of fresh coconut water
- 150 g frozen blackcurrant (thawed or fresh)
- One large-sized green apple (chopped and cored)

- One cup kale (steamed lightly)
- One cup of ice cubes

Method:

1. Take a blender and add green apple, kale, avocado, blackcurrant, and coconut water to it. Blend the mixture and add honey to it.

2. Whizz the smoothie until properly smooth.

3. Divide the smoothie in tall glasses.

4. Serve the smoothie with a green apple from the top. Dust off wheatgrass according to your choice.

Notes:

- In case you do not have wheatgrass, you can use milled flaxseeds in place of it.

- This smoothie comes with a high percentage of magnesium and can be categorized within the group of superfood smoothies.

- You can maintain the proper health of your nervous system with this smoothie.

Matcha Green Smoothie

Total Prep & Cooking Time: 4 minutes

Yields: 2 Servings

Nutrition Facts: Calories: 165 | Protein: 7g | Fat: 6g |

Carbs: 30g | Fiber: 5g

Ingredients:

- Two bananas (frozen)

- One large–sized mango (frozen or fresh)

- Two tsps. of matcha green tea (powder)

- Two cups of baby spinach

- One cup of almond milk (unsweetened)

- 1/3 cup of sliced almonds

- One tsp. of sweetener

- One cup plain Greek yogurt

Method:

1. Take a blender and add all the ingredients to it. Blend the ingredients for about 1 minute to make the mixture smooth.

2. In case you want to add thickness to the smoothie, add ice cubes according to your need. If you want to lower the consistency of the smoothie, add almond milk and blend.

3. Pour the smoothie in tall glasses and enjoy chilled. You can add paper straws for making it look aesthetic.

Notes:

- You can also use coconut milk, cashew milk, rice milk, soy milk, or even unsweetened plain milk in place of almond milk.

- The protein content of the smoothie can be boosted up by adding protein powder to the smoothie.

- You can have a blast of energy after having this smoothie.

- You can experiment with the smoothie by adding fruits of your choice if you want. In case you do not want to use sweetener for the smoothie, try using honey for adding sweetness to it.

Kale and Melon Smoothie

Total Prep & Cooking Time: 12 minutes

Yields: 2 Servings

Nutrition Facts: Calories: 90 | Protein: 4g | Fat: 1.5g | Carbs: 23g | Fiber: 5g

Ingredients:

- One cup of ice cubes
- Two cups of honeydew melon (cubed)
- One cup fresh kale (chopped)
- One medium-sized apple (peeled and cubed)
- One tbsp. fresh lemon juice

Method:

1. Add honeydew melon and ice cubes to a blender and make a fine puree.

2. Add kale, lemon juice, and apple to the melon mixture.

3. Blend all the ingredients properly until smooth. You can add water for adjusting the consistency if needed.

4. Blend again if water is added.

5. Pour the smoothie into two tall glasses.

6. Serve immediately.

Notes:

- This smoothie can be enjoyed during the summer days as it is rich in potassium, vitamin C, and also vitamin B6. It can help a lot in boosting the metabolic rate of the body.

- It comes with a great amount of fiber that can help in maintaining healthy body weight.

- For enhancing the goodness of the smoothie, you can add chia seeds to it.

- If you want the smoothie a bit sweet, you can add frozen bananas to the smoothie.

- This smoothie can help in keeping you hydrated in warm weather.

- The leftover smoothie can be stored in the freezer for two days.

Tropical Kale Carrot Juice

Total Prep & Cooking Time: 12 minutes

Yields: 2 Servings

Nutrition Facts: Calories: 292 | Protein: 4g | Fat: 0.6g | Carbs: 70g | Fiber: 8g

Ingredients:

- Ten medium-sized carrots
- Two fresh oranges
- One bunch kale
- One large apple
- Two pineapple rounds (one-inch thick)

Method:

1. Wash the veggies and fruits properly and dry them—size apple, carrots, and kale by cutting them for fitting them properly in the juicer. For the orange, peel out the skin and cut them into pieces according to the size of the juicer.

2. Process juice from the fruits and veggies properly with the help of a juicer. Make sure that you stir the fruit and vegetable mixture using a spoon for ensuring that the mixture is thorough and smooth.

3. Pour the juice into two juice glasses. Serve them immediately.

Notes:

- This juice can provide you with minerals and vitamins of various types.

- You can boost the performance of your immune system with the help of this juice. It can also be consumed for preventing autoimmune diseases.

- The level of your energy, along with nutrition, can be improved with the consumption of this juice. It can make you feel refreshed and can also improve your level of concentration.

Cranberry Kale Smoothie

Total Prep & Cooking Time: 6 minutes

Yields: 2 servings

Nutrition Facts: Calories: 60 | Carbs: 12g | Protein: 2g | Fat: 1g | Fiber: 4g

Ingredients:

- One cup kale
- One large-sized orange

Half cup of each:

- Water
- Cranberries
- One banana (frozen)

Method:

1. Start by arranging all the required ingredients in one place so that there is no need of rushing for any one of them at the time of blending. Make sure that you cut down the ingredients into smaller sizes so that they can be easily accommodated in the blender. Blend all the ingredients until the smoothie is smooth and is mixed properly.

2. Divide the smoothie into tall glasses and serve immediately.

Grapefruit Celery Juice

Total Prep & Cooking Time: 8 minutes

Yields: 1 Serving

Nutrition Facts: Calories: 53 | Protein: 2g | Fat: 0g | Carbs: 15g | Fiber: 3g

Ingredients:

- One lime
- One cup of ice cubes
- One pomelo grapefruit
- One medium–sized cucumber
- One small apple

Method:

1. Start by washing all the ingredients properly.

2. Peel the outer skin of lime and grapefruit. You can leave the outer skin as it is for making them taste less bitter.

3. Take a juicer and make a juice of all the listed ingredients.

4. Use a blender for blending ice cubes with the juice. Make a smooth mixture and serve immediately.

Notes:

- In case you cannot find pomelo grapefruit in the market, you can use yellow or ruby grapefruit in place of it, orange in place of apple, celeriac root, or zucchini in place of celery and cucumber, and lemon in place of lime.

- You can consume this juice daily for boosting the levels of your immune system.

- As you add pomelo grapefruit and lime to the juice, it will add a sour taste to the juice. Thus, you can have this juice during the hot summer days to get relief from the excess heat.

Cucumber Pineapple Juice

Total Prep & Cooking Time: 10 minutes

Yields: 2 servings

Nutrition Facts: Calories: 75 | Carbs: 16.9g | Protein: 0.9g | Fat: 0.2g | Fiber: 5.9g

Ingredients:

- Two cucumbers (medium-sized)
- Five sticks of fresh celery
- Half fruit of pineapple (outer skin removed)
- Two to three inches of fresh ginger (add more according to taste)
- One lemon

Method:

1. Take all the listed ingredients in a juicer and blend them.

2. Cut the lemon and cucumber into small-sized cubes for fitting them in the juicer. As you cut down the ingredients, it will make the task of blending a lot easier for you and will take less time as well.

3. Make sure you check the consistency of the juice and add water if necessary.

4. Pour the juice equally in two glasses and enjoy!

Notes:

- Cucumber comes with zero fat and is low in calories as well. So, if you are willing to shed your extra body weight, adding cucumber to your daily diet and juices is a great option. In case you do not want to have cucumber as juice, you can include it in your salad.

- Pineapple juice can help a lot in reducing belly fat. Pineapple juice comes with an enzyme named Bromelain that helps in cutting down the excess belly fat. It can also help in easy digestion of proteins.

Summer Blackcurrant Smoothie

Total Prep & Cooking Time: 10 minutes

Yields: 1 Serving

Nutrition Facts: Calories: 228 | Protein: 5g | Fat: 13.5g

| Carbs: 8.9g | Fiber: 8.4g

Ingredients:

Half cup of each:

- Water

- Blackcurrant (frozen or fresh)

- One-fourth cup of strawberries (frozen or fresh)

- Two tbsps. chia seeds (powdered or whole)

- One cup of coconut milk

- Half tsp. vanilla extract (sugar-free)

- Liquid stevia (optional)

Method:

1. Take all the ingredients and put them into a blender. Start by pulsing all the listed ingredients for making a smooth mixture.

2. Leave the pulsed mixture for about 5 minutes.

3. Add vanilla extract to the mixture and blend again.

4. Pour the smoothie into glasses and enjoy!

Notes:

- You can use heavy whipping cream in place of coconut milk.

- Vanilla bean seeds can also be used instead of vanilla extract.

Banana Matcha Smoothie

Total Prep & Cooking Time: 10 minutes

Yields: 1 Serving

Nutrition Facts: Calories: 205 | Protein: 4.2g | Fat: 4g | Carbs: 40g | Fiber: 7g

Ingredients:

- One cup frozen banana (sliced)
- One tsp. matcha green tea powder
- Two tsps. flax seed
- One cup spinach (fresh)
- One tsp. vanilla extract
- One cup of almond milk (unsweetened)

Method:

1. Take all the listed ingredients and place them in a blender. Blend the mixture until smooth.

2. Pour the smoothie in a tall glass and serve immediately. Enjoy!

Notes:

- This banana smoothie comes with the goodness of iron as it includes spinach in it.

- All the ingredients that are used for this smoothie comes with various types of healthy nutrients along with great taste. A banana will provide sweetness, flax seeds will provide fiber, almond milk will lend the smoothness, and matcha green tea powder comes with caffeine.

Simple Celery Cucumber Green Juice

Total Prep & Cooking Time: 20 minutes

Yields: 2 Servings

Nutrition Facts: Calories: 94 | Protein: 2.9g | Fat: 0.9g |

Carbs: 22g | Fiber: 6g

Ingredients:

- Five celery stalks (trimmed ends)

- One medium–sized cucumber (English)

- One bunch fresh kale

- One large apple

- One inch ginger (peeled and fresh)

- Half cup parsley (fresh)

Method:

1. Start by preparing all the listed veggies after washing all of them thoroughly. You will need to cut the vegetables in chunks.

2. Follow this order for placing the veggies in the blender– kale, apple, ginger, parsley, cucumber.

3. Blend all the ingredients properly for making a smooth juice.

4. Divide the juice into two tall glasses.

5. Serve it immediately and enjoy.

Notes:

- Try to make a thick type of juice while using the blender.

- For getting smooth juice, you can use a fine mesh for sieving the prepared juice through the mesh. You will need to press the blended pulp through the mesh for extracting the maximum amount of juice from the remaining pulp.

- You can change the consistency of the juice by adding water or ice.

- For adding a little bit of sweetness, you can use honey.

Spinach, Date, And Vanilla Smoothie

Total Prep & Cooking Time: 8 minutes

Yields: 2 Servings

Nutrition Facts: Calories: 191 | Protein: 3.5g | Fat: 2.8g | Carbs: 42.9g | Fiber: 4.8g

Ingredients:

- One banana (large)
- Two cups of almond milk (vanilla, unsweetened)
- Two cups of spinach
- 4 – 5 Medjool dates(chopped and pitted)

Method:

1. Take a blender and put in all the listed ingredients. Blend for making a smooth mixture.

2. You will need to ensure that there are no existing flecks of spinach or minute pieces of dates. You will need to mix all the ingredients with proper care for getting a perfectly blended smoothie.

3. Pour the smoothie in glasses and enjoy!

Notes:

- If you want the smoothie chilled, you can add in cubes of ice at the time of blending.

- Yogurt can be added to improve the consistency of the smoothie.

- You can experiment with the flavors of the smoothie by adding various types of fruits such as peach, mango, and others as per your choice.

- For improving the nutrient content of the smoothie, add chia seeds, flax seeds, protein powder, and honey. The taste will depend on you.

Kale And Chicken Curry

Total Prep & Cooking Time: 2 hours

Yields: 4 Servings

Nutrition Facts: Calories: 317 | Protein: 25g | Fat: 20g | Carbs: 7g | Fiber: 2.2g

Ingredients:

- Two cardamom pods
- Three garlic cloves
- Two finely chopped chili (bird's eye chili)
- 500 g chicken thighs (boneless and skinned)
- Four cups stock of chicken
- One can tomato (chopped)
- Two onions (diced)
- Two tbsps. of olive oil

One tbsp. of each:

- Curry powder

- Ginger (chopped)

- Six cups of water (boiled)

- Three tbsps. ground turmeric

- 200 ml of light coconut milk

- Half cup kale

Method:

1. Start by placing the chicken in a bowl and add in one tbsp of olive oil. Add one tbsp. of turmeric as well. Mix the chicken properly and leave it to marinate for about half an hour. You will need to mix the chicken with the help of a spoon as otherwise, turmeric can stain your fingers.

2. Take a skillet and heat it over medium flame. Add the marinated chicken and fry it for five minutes or until it gets browned all over. Make sure that the chicken is evenly cooked. Remove the skillet from the heat and keep it aside.

3. Take a frying pan and heat the rest of the olive oil over medium flame. Once the oil gets hot, add chili, garlic, ginger, and onion. Fry the mixture for about ten minutes or until soft.

4. Add curry powder to the onion mixture along with one more tbsp. of turmeric. Cook for 3 – 4 minutes on medium flame.

5. Add chicken stock, tomatoes, cardamom pods, and coconut milk to the pan. Leave the mixture on low flame to simmer for half an hour.

6. Once the sauce gets reduced a bit, add the cooked chicken to the pan along with kale. Cook

the chicken until it mixes well with the sauce, and the kale turns tender.

7. Serve the cooked chicken with rice or buckwheat. In case you are using buckwheat, you will need to simmer it for a small amount of time to prevent it from getting soggy.

8. Garnish by using chopped coriander from the top before serving.

Notes:

- Using turmeric in the chicken curry can help in adding an earthy taste to the dish.

- It can help in activating some particular types of proteins and also protects the body from the onset of excessive stress.

- It helps in enhancing the capability of burning excess fats in the body. The metabolic rate can also be improved.

Tuna, Tomato, And Cucumber Salad

Total Prep & Cooking Time: 30 minutes

Yields: 1 serving

Nutrition Facts: Calorie: 208.9 | Carb: 12g | Protein: 38g | Fat: 2g | Fiber: 2.5g

Ingredients:

- Six oz. Tuna fish
- One cup cherry tomatoes (you can add more if you want)
- Two black peppercorns (ground fresh)
- One lemon
- Two large-sized cucumbers
- Baby arugula or salad greens (according to your preference)

Method:

1. Wash the tomatoes properly and remove the stems. You will need to wash them thoroughly under cold running water. Clean each tomato and dry them with the use of a kitchen towel by patting gently. Slice the tomatoes into halves and keep them in the mixing bowl.

2. You will need to follow the same guidelines for the cucumbers as well. Wash the cucumber under running water and pat dry them with the use of a towel. It is important to clean the veggies properly as you will be consuming them raw as a salad.

3. Chop the cucumbers according to your choice and put them in the mixing bowl along with the cherry tomatoes.

4. Combine tomatoes and cucumbers with the use of a spoon. You can use your hand as well for mixing.

5. In this salad, you will be using the fish along with the oil. Add them to the mixing bowl containing cucumbers and tomatoes. Squeeze lemon juice from the top. Add ground peppercorns to the mixing bowl.

6. Mix everything properly in the mixing bowl. Make sure that you mix gently as you will need to keep the tuna chunks as it is and try not to break them. If you are willing to mash the fish chunks, it won't be a great thing for this salad.

7. For seasoning, squeeze few more drops of lemon juice in accordance with your taste. Splash some oil from the top if you want along with a pinch of salt of you think the fish lacks seasoning.

8. The taste of the salad will depend on your choice, and it can be done by altering the ingredients.

9. Transfer the salad from the mixing bowl to a flat dish. You can increase or decrease the size of servings by adding or discarding the individual ingredients.

10. Place the arugula or salads that you like on the plate.

11. You can place the salad as the base and then top the same with the mixture of tuna fish. Serve immediately.

Note: You can store the leftover salad in the refrigerator for about two days.

Tuscan Bean Soup

Total Prep & Cooking Time: 2 hours

Yields: 8 Servings

Nutrition Facts: Calories: 280 | Protein: 15g | Fat: 3g | Carbs: 48g | Fiber: 21g

Ingredients:

- One pound beans (cannellini, dried)
- Two cups of onion (diced)
- Five cups of kale (chopped and fresh)
- Three bay leaves (dried)
- Four tbsps. white wine vinegar
- Two tbsps. extra-virgin olive oil
- One cup of celery (dried)
- Two cups of carrots (dried)

Four cups of each:

- Chicken broth

- Water

- Two tbsps. fresh garlic (minced)

- Two tsps. of salt

- One tsp. fresh rosemary (minced)

- One can of diced tomatoes (a mixture of tomato, basil, oregano, and garlic)

- Ground pepper (according to taste)

- Parmesan rind (optional)

Method:

1. Start by taking the beans and wash them with plain water. Place the washed beans in a bowl. Add two cups of water to the bowl. Leave the beans soaked in water for about 10 to 20 hours at room temperature.

2. Rinse the beans properly and drain the water.

3. Take a large pot and heat it over medium flame. Add oil to the pot.

4. After the oil gets hot, add onion, celery, along with carrots to the pot. Cook for about 10 minutes or until the mixture turns soft.

5. Add garlic to the onion mixture and stir properly. Cook the onion mixture for one more minute until you can smell a fragrance from the mixture.

6. Add water, soaked beans, parmesan rind, bay leaves, and broth to the pot. Stir the mixture properly.

7. Turn the flame to high and allow the mixture to boil by raising the oven temperature.

8. Cook the mixture for about 10 minutes.

9. Lower the flame and cover the pot partially. Simmer the soup for one hour so that the beans turn tender.

10.   Add in kale, rosemary, and tomatoes to the mixture. Stir the mixture properly so that everything gets mixed in the right way—Cook the soup for half an hour by covering the pot partially.

11.   Remove parmesan rind and bay leaves from the soup. Stir the mixture after adding vinegar and salt.

12.   Add pepper according to your taste.

13.   Serve hot.

Notes:

- In case you do not want to use cannellini beans, you can replace the same with great northern beans.

- Adding parmesan rind to the soup can help in adding a savory and subtle flavor. You can make parmesan rind from cheese blocks according to your choice. The remaining block of parmesan can be stored in the refrigerator for about six months.

- The leftover soup can be stored in the freezer for two days.

- You can toast some bread slices and add to the soup for improving the flavor.

Tofu Mushroom Soup

Total Prep & Cooking Time: 40 minutes

Yields: 6 Servings

Nutrition Facts: Calories: 430 | Protein: 25g | Fat: 22g | Carbs: 49g | Fiber: 4g

Ingredients:

- One oz. of dried mushrooms (porcinis)
- One pound shitake mushrooms (fresh)
- One pound cremini or button mushrooms (quartered)
- Two tsps. of salt
- One garlic head (halved)
- Two tbsps. soy sauce
- Five slices of ginger (fresh)

- Fifteen oz. tofu (soft or firm, diced)

- Two tbsps. chives (chopped)

- Half cup of cilantro (chopped)

Method:

1. Take a bowl and place the dried mushrooms. Add two cups of boiling water to the bowl and cover it. Allow the mushrooms to sit for about half an hour. In case the mushrooms are sandy in nature, agitate at regular intervals.

2. Take a strainer and line it with cheesecloth. Place a bowl under the strainer for storing the liquid. Drain the mushroom through the cheesecloth and twist the mushrooms. In this way, you will be able to squeeze out most of the mushroom

juice. You can either discard the squeezed mushrooms or keep it aside for using it for one more time.

3. Take the shitake mushrooms and pull out the stems. Slice the mushrooms caps thinly and keep it aside.

4. Add enough water to the broth of mushroom for making about 8 cups of liquid and add it to a saucepan. Add the stems of shitake mushroom to it along with quartered cremini or button mushrooms, slices of ginger halved garlic head and salt. Bring the mixture to a boil by increasing the flame.

5. Reduce the flame, cover the pot, and simmer it for half an hour.

6. Use a spoon for removing stems, mushrooms, ginger, and garlic from the soup. Add soy sauce to it and add salt according to your taste.

7. Boil the broth once again and start adding cubes of tofu. Reduce the flame and cover the pot partially. Simmer the soup for half an hour. The tofu cubes will puff up a bit. It will become spongy and porous.

8. Add the sliced caps of shitake mushrooms to the soup and simmer for five minutes.

9. Add chives and cilantro to the soup.

10. Check the seasoning of the soup according to your taste and serve hot.

Notes:

• You can replace plain water with chicken stock as well. In case you want to use chicken stock, add cornstarch solution to it. Mix two tbsps. of

water with one tbsp. of cornstarch for making
the solution.

- It is a great family dish and is actually vegan.

- Tofu is made from the curds of soybean. It
  comes with the goodness of special types of
  proteins that can help in lowering the overall risk
  of developing chronic diseases.

- It can help in dealing with low–density
  lipoprotein or LDL cholesterol that is widely
  known as the bad cholesterol.

- The leftover soup can be stored in the
  refrigerator for three to four days. You can add
  toasted breadsticks to the soup.

Veggie Tofu Stir Fry

Total Prep & Cooking Time: 30 minutes

Yields: 4 servings

Nutrition Facts: Calories: 157 | Carbs: 19g | Protein: 6.9g | Fat: 7g | Fiber: 4.5g

Ingredients:

- Two packages of tofu (14 oz. package, do not use silken or firm tofu other than extra-firm one)
- Three tbsps. of soy sauce (low-sodium)
- One tbsp. of grapeseed oil or canola oil
- One bunch green onions (chopped finely)
- Three cloves of garlic (minced, fresh)
- One tbsp. ginger (fresh, minced)

- Two tsps. chili paste (you can replace this with half tsp. of red pepper flakes)

- Ten oz. baby spinach

- Two tsps. of sesame oil

- Two tbsps. sesame seeds (toasted)

For the serving:

- Quinoa

- Cauliflower rice

- Rice o soba noodles

- Brown rice (prepared)

Method:

1. Start by draining the tofu. Wrap the tofu blocks in a layer of paper towel and dry them by

patting. Press the tofu blocks lightly for squeezing out extra moisture. After you are done with drying the tofu, cut them into small cubes of four inches.

2. Take a large skillet and heat it over medium flame. Add canola oil to the skillet. After the oil gets hot, add the tofu cubes. Make sure that the oil is not smoking and be careful while adding tofu cubes to the oil as it can splatter a bit.

3. Drizzle one tbsp. of soy sauce from the top.

4. Sauté the tofu cubes properly and stir them occasionally. Make sure that the tofu cubes are colored nicely on all sides. Cook the cubes until all the moisture is gone, for about ten minutes.

5. Do not stir the tofu cubes continuously. Allowing the cubes to sit on the hot oil for a moment will make them brown.

6. Add two-third of green onion, garlic, chili paste, ginger, and two tbsps. of soy sauce to the skillet. Stir the tofu cubes properly and cook them till fragrant for about one minute.

7. Start adding spinach to the skillet. Stir the spinach until it wilts so that you can add in more spinach to the skillet.

8. After the first batch of spinach has wilted, keep on adding the rest of the spinach until you are done with all the spinach.

9. You might feel that the amount of spinach is excessive at first, but it will wilt down slowly.

10. Add sesame seeds along with the sesame oil.

11. Remove the skillet from the heat.

12. Sprinkle the remaining green onions from the top.

13.   Serve hot with noodles, brown rice, or anything that you feel like.

14.   You can add few dashes of chili flakes or paste along with soy sauce from the top for extra flavor.

Notes:

- You will need to be careful in case you are using olive oil. It can smoke at a lower temperature, and thus the overall chance of burning the food will increase. You will need to save the preparation from getting an awkward flavor by adding only the required amount. Make sure that you check properly every time at the time of adding oil.

- You can use other types of leaves in place of spinach that you have in the freezer. Spinach is most widely used as it can get wilted very easily. So, you can cook the tofu properly without any extra time. For example, if you use other types of vegetables such as broccoli or peppers, you will need to keep the cooked tofu aside after step 3. Add a few more drops of oil along with garlic and ginger if you want. Add veggies of your choice to the pan. Cook the vegetables properly for making them tender. You will need to cook them for about 8 – 10 minutes, depending on the type of vegetable that you will be using. Add cooked tofu to the pan and continue with the rest of the recipe.

- You can store the dish in the refrigerator for later use. You can store it for about five days. For consuming the leftover dish, place the dish in a microwave oven for reheating.

Shrimp Arugula Salad

Total Prep & Cooking Time: 15 minutes

Yields: 4 Servings

Nutrition Facts: Calories: 340 | Protein: 27g | Fat: 25g | Carbs: 11g | Fiber: 5.2g

Ingredients:

- Two lemons (one for wedges and the other for juice)
- One large avocado (sliced)
- Ten cups arugula (baby arugula)
- One pound shrimp (large-sized, cooked)
- Sea salt
- Five tbsps. olive oil (extra-virgin)
- Pepper (for seasoning, cracked and fresh)

Method:

1. Start by preparing a mixture of arugula, avocado, and cooked shrimp in a mixing bowl.

2. Add lemon juice, three tbsps. of olive oil, pepper, and salt for adding taste to the mixture. You can alter the proportions according to your taste.

3. You can add more olive oil after tossing the mixture if needed. You will need to coat the arugula with oil. Adjust the mixture seasoning after tasting.

4. Place wedges of lemon on the sides at the time of serving.

Notes:

- If you do not want to use avocado, you can use shaved parmesan.

- This recipe is low in carbs and is perfect for maintaining healthy body weight.

- You can include this salad for your daily lunch.

- The leftover salad can be stored in the freezer for two days for later use.

Buckwheat Noodles With King Prawn

Total Prep & Cooking Time: 30 minutes

Yields: 4 servings

Nutrition Facts: Calories: 423 | Carbs: 45g | Protein: 20.5g | Fat: 18g | Fiber: 0.5g

Ingredients:

- 300 g soba noodles or buckwheat noodles (100% buckwheat will work the best)
- One large red onion (sliced thin)
- Two tbsps. olive oil (extra–virgin)
- Three celery sticks (chopped)

100 g of each:

- Green beans (chopped)
- Kale (chopped)

- Three cloves of garlic (chopped finely or grated)

- Three cm of fresh ginger (grated)

- Two tbsps. soy sauce or tamari sauce

- Three tbsps. parsley (chopped)

- 700 g king prawns

- One bird's eye chili (seeds removed, finely

  chopped)

Method:

1. Take a pan and heat it on medium flame. Put the

   noodles in the pan and cook it for five to six

   minutes or until you think it is perfect. Wash the

   cooked noodles thoroughly under running water

   and make sure that the water is cold. Add olive

   oil to the noodles and mix it properly. This is

   necessary so that the noodles do not stick to

   each other. Cover the noodles and keep it aside.

2. While the noodles are being cooked in the pan, try to arrange all the ingredients on your countertop so that there is no wastage of time.

3. Take a large frying pan and heat it over medium flame. Add olive oil to the pan and allow the oil to get hot. Start adding celery and red onions to the pan. Stir the veggies gently for three to four minutes or until they become tender. Add beans and kale to the onion mixture and mix everything properly on a medium flame for about three minutes.

4. Lower the flame and start adding the remaining ingredients to the pan. Add king prawns, garlic, chili, and ginger to the pan. Keep frying the ingredients in the pan until the prawns turn light brown in color. It will take somewhat around three to four minutes for the color to appear on the prawns.

5. After the prawns are nicely browned, add cooked noodles to the pan and mix well.

6. Add the sauce to the noodles and sauté properly for two to three minutes.

7. Serve the noodles on a plate and top it with parsley from the top.

Sesame Chicken Salad

Total Prep & Cooking Time: 40 minutes

Yields: 4 Servings

Nutrition Facts: Calories: 350 | Protein: 33g | Fat: 19g | Carbs: 11g | Fiber: 4.2g

Ingredients:

- Two pounds of chicken thighs (skinless and boneless)
- Two cups carrots (cut into matchsticks or shredded)
- One cup almond (sliced)
- One cup cilantro (chopped roughly)
- Five green onions (diced)
- Two tbsps. black sesame seeds

- One tbsp. of white sesame seeds

- One can mandarin oranges (with no syrup or sugar)

- One small red cabbage (sliced thinly)

- One small green cabbage (sliced thinly)

For the dressing:

- One cup coconut amino

- Four tbsps. avocado oil

- Two tbsps. of sesame oil (toasted)

- One tbsp. of fresh ginger (minced)

  One tsp. of onion powder

- Two tsps. salt

- One tsp. pepper

- One cup of red wine vinegar

Method:

1. Take a large mixing bowl for preparing the salad.

2. Prepare the dressing by mixing all the ingredients.

3. Use a plastic bag for coating the chicken thighs with four tbsps. of the prepared dressing.

4. Allow the chicken to marinate for about two to three hours.

5. Take a skillet and heat it over medium flame. Place the marinated chicken on the skillet and grill the chicken for about ten minutes on medium flame. Make sure that both sides of the chicken are grilled properly.

6. Remove the chicken from the pan and allow it to cool at room temperature. After the chicken

cools down, chop it down for mixing with the salad.

7. Prepare the salad in a mixing bowl. Add the cooked chicken to the salad and mix it properly.

8. Add dressing at the end and toss the salad for even coating of the dressing.

9. Serve with lunch or dinner.

Notes:

- In case you do not want to use red wine vinegar, you can replace it with apple cider vinegar. It will provide the same taste.

- You can store the leftover salad in the refrigerator for two days for using later.

Spicy Chickpea Stew With Baked Potatoes

Total Prep & Cooking Time: 1 hour 20 minutes

Yields: 4 Servings

Nutrition Facts: Calories: 348.5 | Protein: 7.5g | Fat: 16.7g | Carbs: 41.8g | Fiber: 5.9g

Ingredients:

- Six to seven baking potatoes (make sure you prick the potatoes all over)
- Two large red onions (chopped finely)
- Two tbsps. olive oil (extra-virgin)
- Five cloves of fresh garlic (crushed or grated)
- Two tbsps. cumin seeds
- Two tsps. chili flakes (you can reduce or add according to your taste)

- Two cm fresh ginger (grated)

- One cup of water

- Two tbsps. turmeric

- Two cans of tomatoes (chopped)

- Two cans of chickpeas (you can use kidney beans as well)

- Three tbsps. cocoa powder (unsweetened)

- Three tbsps. parsley (chopped)

- Two large yellow peppers (chopped)

- Pepper and salt (according to taste)

Optional: Side salad

Method:

1. Start by preheating the oven to 250 degrees Celsius. You can start preparing the rest of the ingredients.

2. When the oven turns hot, add the baking potatoes to the oven and cook them for about one hour or until they are ready as you like them. In case you do not have an oven, you can use the traditional way of baking potatoes.

3. After you are done with placing the potatoes in the oven, take a saucepan and heat it over medium flame. Add olive oil to the pan and wait for it to get hot.

4. Add onion to the pan and cook it gently. Cook the onions for about five minutes or until the onions turn soft. Make sure that you do not brown the onions.

5. Add ginger, garlic, chili, and cumin to the pan—
   Cook for one more minute on low flame. Add
   turmeric to the onion mixture along with a
   gentle splash of water.

6. Cook the onions for one more minute and make
   sure that the pan does not get excessively dry.

7. Add cocoa powder, tomatoes, yellow pepper, and
   chickpeas to the pan. Bring the mixture to a boil
   and then simmer it for about 50 minutes on low
   flame. You will have to make the sauce turn
   thick.

8. Add two tbsps. of parsley from the top and give
   the stew a stir. Add pepper and salt according to
   your taste.

9. Place the baked potatoes on a plate and serve it
   with the stew from the top. You can serve the
   same with a very simple side salad as well.

Notes:

- You can use kidney beans in place of chickpeas.

- If you do not want to use yellow peppers, you can use peppers of any color.

- Cocoa powder can be replaced with cacao.

- If you want, the water of chickpeas can be added to the chickpeas.

Prawn Arrabbiata

Total Prep & Cooking Time: 30 minutes

Yields: 2 Servings

Nutrition Facts: Calories: 426 | Protein: 34g | Fat: 25.6g | Carbs: 20.8g | Fiber: 7g

Ingredients:

- One large onion (diced finely)
- Four tbsps. olive oil (extra-virgin)
- Four cloves of garlic (diced finely)
- Half tsp. of chili flakes
- One tsp. of salt
- Two zucchinis (medium-sized, ribbon-shaped or noodles)
- Two cup tomatoes (tinned and chopped)

- One red pepper (diced)

- One cup parmesan cheese (grated)

- 300 g shrimp or prawn (large-sized, peeled, and raw)

- Basil or parsley (for garnishing, optional)

Method:

1. Take the zucchini and use a veggie spiralizer or peeler for making spirals of zucchini. In case you do not have a peeler or spiralizer, you can make just the zucchini in simple strips.

2. Take a skillet and heat it over medium flame. Add one tbsp. of olive oil to the skillet and allow it to get hot. Add prawns to the skillet and fry them for about three to four minutes. Stir the prawns occasionally and transfer them to a bowl.

3. Heat a pan over medium flame and add two tbsps. of olive oil. Add onion and pepper to the pan and sauté them for about four minutes. Cook until the onions turn tender and light brown in color.

4. Stir the onion mixture after adding salt, garlic, and chili.

5. Add tomatoes to the pan and mix properly.

6. Set the flame at low and cook the onion mixture for two minutes.

7. In case the tomatoes turn out to be dry in the pan, you can add a splash of water.

8. Add prawn and zucchini noodles to the pan and mix them thoroughly.

9. Keep on mixing for about two minutes. Make sure that the zucchini does not get extremely

tender. In case the zucchini gets tender, it will turn out to be soggy.

10.   Serve the dish in a bowl and top it with cheese. Add fresh basil or parsley for garnishing.

Notes:

- You can opt for aged cheddar in place of grated parmesan. In case you are allergic to prawns, you can replace the same with diced chicken— Cook the diced chicken for five minutes before adding to the salad.

- The zucchini noodles can be replaced with sweet potato salad if you want to. You can also opt for low-carb spaghetti-like shirataki noodles or konjac noodles.

- The leftover dish can be stored in the freezer for one day for consuming later.

- If you want the dish to be a bit spicy, add chili flakes from the top.

The Sirtfood Shakshuka

Total Prep & Cooking Time: 50 minutes

Yields: 4 Servings

Nutrition Facts: Calories: 152 | Protein: 10g | Fat: 9g | Carbs: 17g | Fiber: 4g

Ingredients:

- 50 g red onion (chopped finely)

- One tbsp. olive oil (extra-virgin)

- 40 g celery (chopped finely)

- One clove of fresh garlic (chopped finely)

- One bird's eye chili (chopped finely)

One tsp. of each:

- Turmeric (ground)

- Cumin (ground)

- Two tsps. paprika

- 500 g tomatoes (tinned and chopped)

- 40 g kale (chopped roughly, stems removed)

- Two large eggs

- Two tbsps. parsley (chopped)

Method

1. Take a large frying pan and heat it over medium flame. Add olive oil to the pan and allow it to get hot. Make sure that it does not smoke.

2. Add chili, onion, celery, garlic, and spices to the pan—Fry the spice mixture for about two minutes.

3. Add chopped tomatoes to the pan and simmer the mixture for half an hour. Ensure that you stir the mixture properly.

4. Add kale to the mixture and cook the mixture for five more minutes.

5. You can adjust the consistency of the mixture by adding a splash of water if you do not want the mixture to be thick.

6. After you are satisfied with the mixture consistency, add chopped parsley to the mixture.

7. Stir the mixture properly to ensure that everything gets mixed properly.

8. Make two wells in the mixture and crack the eggs in them.

9. Set the flame to low and cook the shakshuka for about 12 minutes by covering the pan with a lid. Make the yolk portion of the egg runny and the white portion firm. In case you want the yolk to be firm, you will need to cook the mixture for 5 more minutes.

10.   Serve the dish directly from the pan.

Sirtfood Bites

Total Prep & Cooking Time: 15 minutes

Yields: 20 bites (approx)

Nutrition Facts: Calories: 237 | Protein: 5g | Fat: 11.5g | Carbs: 30g | Fiber: 3g

Ingredients:

- One tbsp. of olive oil (extra-virgin)

- 300 g Medjool dates (peeled)

- 200 g walnuts

- Two tbsps. of turmeric (ground)

- Half tbsp. cocoa powder

- 1/3 tsp. vanilla extract

- 40 g dark chocolate (broken)

- Water

Method:

- Take a food processor and add broken pieces of dark chocolate to it. Process the chocolate and make a fine powder.

- Add all the ingredients in the food processor. Do not add water.

- Blend all the ingredients properly.

- After you are done with blending, take out the mixture and start making small balls from the mixture.

- In case the mixture gets stuck to your hands, you can add a bit of water for maintaining the consistency of the chocolate mixture.

- After you have prepared all the balls, place them in an air-tight container. Keep the container in the freezer for about one hour.

- You can add extra flavor to the bites by rolling them in desiccated coconut before putting them in the freezer.

- You can serve the bites with chocolate syrup from the top (optional). The leftover bites can be stored in the freezer for about one week.

Notes:

- If you do not want to use vanilla extract for the bites, you can use vanilla pods. Scrape the seeds out of the pod for use in the dish.

- You can replace the dark chocolate with cocoa nibs.

Choco Chip Granola

Total Prep & Cooking Time: 40 minutes

Yields: 12 Servings

Nutrition Facts: Calories: 240 | Protein: 5.5g | Fat: 11g | Carbs: 30g | Fiber: 3g

Ingredients:

- One cup peanut butter (salted and creamy)
- Half cup olive oil
- Three tbsps. sugar (organic)
- One-quarter cup of maple syrup
- Oat cups (rolled)
- One cup choco chips (bittersweet or dark and dairy-free)

Method:

1. Start by setting the oven temperature to 350 degrees Fahrenheit. Preheat the oven.

2. Take a large mixing bowl and mix oats and sugar.

3. Take a small frying pan and heat it over medium flame. Add peanut butter, olive oil, and maple syrup to the pan and mix them. You will need to warm them properly. Make sure that the consistency of the mixture is perfect.

4. Add the peanut butter mixture to the mixing bowl over the mixture of oats. Stir the mixture properly for ensuring proper mixing. You can add in more oats to the mixture if you think that the mixture is excessively wet.

5. Take a baking sheet for spreading out the mixture evenly. Place the baking sheet and place it in the oven. Bake it for about 25 minutes or until they turn golden brown in color all over.

6. For ensuring even baking, you will need to toss them once after the mark of 15 minutes.

7. Take out the tray and toss it once for reducing the heat. Leave it aside for cooling down completely.

8. Take a mixing bowl or a storage container and pour the mixture into it. Shake or stir them after you have added the choco chips.

9. The granola can be enjoyed with almond milk or other things of your choice.

10. The granola can be stored in the freezer for about two weeks to keep them fresh and tasty.

Notes:

- Olive oil can be replaced with melted coconut oil or even avocado oil according to your choice.

- In case you are not vegan, you can use honey. Agave nectar can also be used in place of maple syrup.

Pecan Pie Bites

Total Prep & Cooking Time: 20 minutes

Yields: 10 Servings

Nutrition Facts: Calories: 122 | Protein: 1.5g | Fat: 6.9g | Carbs: 17g | Fiber: 2.5g

Ingredients:

- One tsp. of sea salt
- Half tsp. vanilla extract (pure)
- One cup of dates (packed and soft pitted)
- Half cup pecans

Method:

- Take a food processor and process all the ingredients.

- In order to make the perfect dough, you will need to maintain proper consistency.

- Pour the mixture from the processor on a mixing bowl. Start making small balls from the dough after rolling them once.

- Refrigerate the pecan bites for using them later.

Notes:

- Dates can be digested very easily and also comes with the goodness of dietary fiber. It can also help in controlling the level of blood sugar.

- In case you do not want to use pecans, you can use walnuts. Dates can be replaced with raisins.

- For developing better flavor, add a pinch of cinnamon, nutmeg, and ginger. It will help in adding an extra flavor to the bites.

- For making the dates soft, take a bowl of water and soak the dates in it. Drain the dates after 15 minutes.

- If you are going to use raisins in place of dates, make sure that you soak them for about 15 minutes in hot water. You will need to cut the raisins in structures of a bar shape.

Buckwheat Crackers

Total Prep & Cooking Time: 1 hour

Yields: 40 crackers

Nutrition Facts: Calories: 290 | Protein: 7g | Fat: 13g | Carbs: 35.5g | Fiber: 5g

Ingredients:

- One cup plain water
- Two large sweet potatoes (grated)
- Two cups buckwheat groats
- Half tsp. sea salt
- Seven tbsps. olive oil (extra-virgin)
- One cup sesame seeds
- Half cup flax seeds (organic)

Method:

1. Before starting with the recipe, soak the buckwheat groats for about four hours.

2. Soak the flax seeds in water for about 10 minutes so that they turn into a jelly-like substance after soaking in water.

3. Grate the sweet potatoes and make a mixture in a bowl with all the ingredients.

4. Use a parchment paper for flat spreading the mixture. Cover the layer of the mixture with another parchment paper.

5. With the help of a rolling pin, press the mixture layer and sprinkle sesame seeds from the top.

6. Set the oven temperature to 300 degrees Fahrenheit and preheat. Bake the mixture layer

in the oven for about 20 minutes for making the crackers.

7. Take out the crackers from the oven and cut them into square-shape with the help of a pizza cutter or a knife.

8. Set the temperature of the oven to 250 degrees Fahrenheit and bake the crackers once again for half an hour for making them crisp and dry.

Notes:

• Permit the buckwheat groats to stay intact after soaking. You can also make a paste by blending the groats before the process of baking. The option that you will be choosing will depend on your convenience.

- As you will be rolling the mixture with a rolling pin, roll the layer gently so that that the sesame seeds can get stuck to the upper layer.

- After taking out the crackers from the oven, allow them to cool and handle with care. They can break very if handled roughly.

- In case you want crispier crackers, you will need to roll the dough thinner,

- The crackers can be stored in the refrigerator for five days. Store them in an air-tight container.

CHAPTER 12: WARNINGS

The sirtfood diet is a completely new concept in the world of dieting. So, there are certain things that you will need to take into consideration before opting for the diet plan. The first phase of the diet is actually very low in calories and is also insufficient nutritionally. There are no forms of security issues for any healthy average adult to think about the brief duration of the diet. But, for some people, who are suffering from diabetes, the limitation of calories and also living only on the green juice for the first few days might result in triggering unsafe alterations in the levels of blood sugar.

Not only that, but a healthy person can also experience some of the side effects. In most of the cases, the problem comes with the appetite. Consuming only about 1000 – 1500 calories every day can leave anyone starving, especially all that you will be taking is green juice. The green juice is low in fiber content, which is the nutrient responsible for making you feel full. All throughout the course of phase one, you might also experience other side effects like irritation, fatigue, and also lightheadedness because of the calorie limitation. Otherwise, if the diet plan is followed for three weeks, only any major health repercussions are very unlikely. The sirtdiet is all about low calories, and the first phase is not at all balanced nutritionally. It can even leave you starving. It is better to consult with your doctor first before opting for the die.

CONCLUSION

Thank you for making it through to the end of *The Sirtfood Diet*, let's hope it was informative and able to provide you with all of the tools you need to achieve your goals whatever they may be.

This book is all about the great roles that are played by the sirtuins in sirtdiet. The scientific processes behind the functioning of the diet have also been explained. Now, your job is to start following the diet, taking into consideration any kind of health issue. The list of sirtfoods consists of major food items from our daily lives. Sirtfood can effectively activate the sirtuins that can help in losing a great deal of body weight. You will need to maintain the diet during the two phases that last for three weeks. The main aim will be to lower down the consumption of calories. Detailed information about both phases of the diet has been provided in this book.

Sirtuins not only help in losing weight but also comes with other benefits when it is about the reduction of inflammation. As you follow the diet, you will be able to maintain the health of your heart along with the prevention of the development of tumors. Losing weight cannot be achieved overnight, and you will need to wait for the results. For that, you will need to consume sirtfoods in your daily diet after the phases of the sirtdiet are over. You can prepare some tasty meals from the recipes provided.

Finally, if you found this book useful in any way, a review on Amazon is always appreciated!

CPSIA information can be obtained
at www.ICGtesting.com
Printed in the USA
BVHW060834050421
604216BV00017B/773

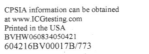

9 781802 218800